Clinical Advances in Cerebral Aneurysm Treatment

Clinical Advances in Cerebral Aneurysm Treatment

Editor

Ramazan Jabbarli

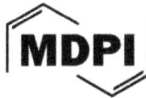

Basel • Beijing • Wuhan • Barcelona • Belgrade • Novi Sad • Cluj • Manchester

Editor
Ramazan Jabbarli
University Hospital Essen
Essen
Germany

Editorial Office
MDPI
St. Alban-Anlage 66
4052 Basel, Switzerland

This is a reprint of articles from the Special Issue published online in the open access journal *Journal of Clinical Medicine* (ISSN 2077-0383) (available at: https://www.mdpi.com/journal/jcm/special_issues/PT2DM24OFA).

For citation purposes, cite each article independently as indicated on the article page online and as indicated below:

Lastname, A.A.; Lastname, B.B. Article Title. *Journal Name* **Year**, *Volume Number*, Page Range.

ISBN 978-3-7258-1213-4 (Hbk)
ISBN 978-3-7258-1214-1 (PDF)
doi.org/10.3390/books978-3-7258-1214-1

© 2024 by the authors. Articles in this book are Open Access and distributed under the Creative Commons Attribution (CC BY) license. The book as a whole is distributed by MDPI under the terms and conditions of the Creative Commons Attribution-NonCommercial-NoDerivs (CC BY-NC-ND) license.

Contents

Ramazan Jabbarli
Addressing Challenges in Cerebral Aneurysm Management: Strategies to Enhance Patient Outcomes
Reprinted from: *J. Clin. Med.* **2024**, *13*, 2308, doi:10.3390/jcm13082308 1

Hartmut Vatter, Erdem Güresir, Ralph König, Gregor Durner, Rolf Kalff, Patrick Schuss, et al.
Invasive Diagnostic and Therapeutic Management of Cerebral VasoSpasm after Aneurysmal Subarachnoid Hemorrhage (IMCVS)—A Phase 2 Randomized Controlled Trial
Reprinted from: *J. Clin. Med.* **2022**, *11*, 6197, doi:10.3390/jcm11206197 5

Erdem Güresir, Thomas Welchowski, Tim Lampmann, Simon Brandecker, Agi Güresir, Johannes Wach, et al.
Delayed Cerebral Ischemia after Aneurysmal Subarachnoid Hemorrhage: The Results of Induced Hypertension Only after the IMCVS Trial—A Prospective Cohort Study
Reprinted from: *J. Clin. Med.* **2022**, *11*, 5850, doi:10.3390/jcm11195850 13

Maryam Said, Thiemo Florin Dinger, Meltem Gümüs, Laurèl Rauschenbach, Mehdi Chihi, Jan Rodemerk, et al.
Impact of Anemia Severity on the Outcome of an Aneurysmal Subarachnoid Hemorrhage
Reprinted from: *J. Clin. Med.* **2022**, *11*, 6258, doi:10.3390/jcm11216258 20

Maryam Said, Meltem Gümüs, Jan Rodemerk, Mehdi Chihi, Laurèl Rauschenbach, Thiemo F. Dinger, et al.
Morphometric Study of the Initial Ventricular Indices to Predict the Complications and Outcome of Aneurysmal Subarachnoid Hemorrhage
Reprinted from: *J. Clin. Med.* **2023**, *12*, 2585, doi:10.3390/jcm12072585 33

Diana L. Alsbrook, Mario Di Napoli, Kunal Bhatia, Masoom Desai, Archana Hinduja, Clio A. Rubinos, et al.
Pathophysiology of Early Brain Injury and Its Association with Delayed Cerebral Ischemia in Aneurysmal Subarachnoid Hemorrhage: A Review of Current Literature
Reprinted from: *J. Clin. Med.* **2023**, *12*, 1015, doi:10.3390/jcm12031015 45

Michael Veldeman, Tobias Rossmann, Miriam Weiss, Catharina Conzen-Dilger, Miikka Korja, Anke Hoellig, et al.
Aneurysmal Subarachnoid Hemorrhage in Hospitalized Patients on Anticoagulants—A Two Center Matched Case-Control Study
Reprinted from: *J. Clin. Med.* **2023**, *12*, 1476, doi:10.3390/jcm12041476 62

Marie-Sophie Schüngel, Karl-Titus Hoffmann, Erik Weber, Jens Maybaum, Nikolaos Bailis, Maximilian Scheer, et al.
Distal Flow Diversion with Anti-Thrombotically Coated and Bare Metal Low-Profile Flow Diverters—A Comparison
Reprinted from: *J. Clin. Med.* **2023**, *12*, 2700, doi:10.3390/jcm12072700 74

Johannes Wach, Martin Vychopen, Agi Güresir and Erdem Güresir
Anti-Inflammatory Drug Therapy in Aneurysmal Subarachnoid Hemorrhage: A Systematic Review and Meta-Analysis of Prospective Randomized and Placebo-Controlled Trials
Reprinted from: *J. Clin. Med.* **2023**, *12*, 4165, doi:10.3390/jcm12124165 91

Katarzyna Wójtowicz, Lukasz Przepiorka, Sławomir Kujawski, Andrzej Marchel and Przemysław Kunert
Unruptured Anterior Communicating Artery Aneurysms: Management Strategy and Results of a Single-Center Experience
Reprinted from: *J. Clin. Med.* **2023**, *12*, 4619, doi:10.3390/jcm12144619 . . . . **107**

Katarzyna Wójtowicz, Lukasz Przepiorka, Sławomir Kujawski, Edyta Maj, Andrzej Marchel and Przemysław Kunert
Retrospective Application of Risk Scores to Unruptured Anterior Communicating Artery Aneurysms
Reprinted from: *J. Clin. Med.* **2024**, *13*, 789, doi:10.3390/jcm13030789 . . . . **117**

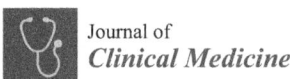 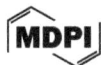

Editorial

Addressing Challenges in Cerebral Aneurysm Management: Strategies to Enhance Patient Outcomes

Ramazan Jabbarli

Department of Neurosurgery & Spine Surgery, University Hospital Essen, 45147 Essen, Germany; ramazan.jabbarli@uk-essen.de

We are pleased to present a Special Issue dedicated to addressing the current challenges in the management of cerebral aneurysms (CA). This Special Issue comprises ten publications covering various topics related to the diagnosis and treatment of CA. A detailed list of contributions is provided at the end of this article.

Cerebral aneurysms (CA) represent saccular or fusiform enlargements of intracranial arterial vasculature, believed to develop under the prolonged influence of multiple endogenous and exogenous factors, the entirety of which remains incompletely elucidated [1]. CA is present in approximately 3% of the adult healthy population as small vascular lesions with an average diameter of 6–7 mm [2,3]. CA typically remains asymptomatic throughout an individual's lifetime. However, the rupture of a CA leads to an aneurysmal subarachnoid hemorrhage (SAH), a devastating form of hemorrhagic stroke associated with high morbidity and mortality rates [4]. A myriad of complications occurring at different stages of SAH significantly contribute to the poor outcomes observed in individuals with ruptured CA [5–7].

Among the various pathophysiologic pathways implicated in CA development, neuro-inflammation is recognized as a key process driving CA genesis [8]. To shed further light on the role of neuro-inflammation in the pathophysiology of CA and its complications, Wach et al. (Contribution 1) conducted a systematic review and meta-analysis focusing on anti-inflammatory drug therapy in SAH. Their findings suggest that anti-inflammatory therapy in SAH patients may improve neurological outcomes without increasing mortality rates. They recommend further investigation through prospective multicenter randomized studies to evaluate the effects of inflammation management in SAH.

Given the poor outcomes associated with SAH, the preventive treatment of rupture-prone CA before the occurrence of a bleeding event is crucial for achieving favorable treatment results [9,10]. However, not all CA ruptures, and there is a significant risk of peri-procedural complications during CA treatment [11]. Thus, the proper identification of rupture-prone CA and the selection of individuals who may benefit from preventive CA treatment pose significant challenges in CA management. To facilitate this selection process, several scores assessing rupture risk have been developed in recent years [12,13]. Two studies by Wójtowicz et al. (Contributions 2 and 3) focused on the challenges in managing unruptured CA, particularly those located at the anterior communicating artery. These studies evaluated long-term functional outcomes following conservative and invasive management approaches and validated the accuracy and clinical applicability of different risk scores in their cohort.

In cases requiring CA treatment, optimizing the treatment process to prevent iatrogenic complications and achieve sustainable treatment outcomes is of paramount importance [10,14]. Endovascular treatment modalities have shown consistent progress over the past three decades, demonstrating improved applicability for various CA locations and morphologies [15]. Shüngel et al. (Contribution 4) present a comparative study on the use of distal flow diversion with anti-thrombotically coated and bare metal low-profile flow diverters in this issue.

Citation: Jabbarli, R. Addressing Challenges in Cerebral Aneurysm Management: Strategies to Enhance Patient Outcomes. *J. Clin. Med.* **2024**, *13*, 2308. https://doi.org/10.3390/jcm13082308

Received: 9 April 2024
Accepted: 11 April 2024
Published: 16 April 2024

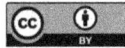

Copyright: © 2024 by the author. Licensee MDPI, Basel, Switzerland. This article is an open access article distributed under the terms and conditions of the Creative Commons Attribution (CC BY) license (https://creativecommons.org/licenses/by/4.0/).

As previously mentioned, SAH poses substantial morbidity and mortality risks despite maximal treatment efforts. Early and delayed complications of SAH, along with its initial severity, are major determinants of patient outcomes [5–7]. This Special Issue focuses particularly on studies addressing different aspects of SAH management, which play crucial roles in patient outcomes. In particular, Alsbrook et al. (Contribution 5) provide a systematic review of the pathophysiological backgrounds, diagnostic approaches, and therapeutic targets for managing early and delayed brain injuries after SAH, emphasizing perspectives for future experimental and clinical research.

The significance of detailed analysis of initial computed tomography scans for predicting complications and outcomes after SAH ([7,16], Contribution 6) is demonstrated in a study by Said et al. (Contribution 6). They show that not only the extent of intracranial bleeding but also the morphology of the ventricular system may serve as valuable radiographic markers for early recognition of complications and poor outcomes in SAH.

The use of anticoagulants before or during SAH can influence treatment outcomes, necessitating a detailed analysis. Veldeman et al. (Contribution 7) compare the impact of direct oral anticoagulants and vitamin K antagonists on the initial clinical and radiographic severity of SAH, as well as patient outcomes.

Güresir et al. (Contribution 8) and Vatter et al. (Contribution 9) present two studies from their center comparing conservative and invasive management options for cerebral vasospasm, addressing different treatment approaches and their effects on the occurrence of delayed cerebral ischemia and poor functional outcomes after SAH.

Proper intensive care management is essential for preventing many complications and irreversible brain damage after CA rupture. Anemia is a common condition following SAH, particularly in severely affected patients during the first weeks after the bleeding event ([17], contribution 10). Despite the lack of specific guidelines for anemia treatment after SAH, its management remains a highly debated topic in intensive care units. To address this issue, Said et al. (Contribution 10) analyze the effect of anemia on the course and outcome of SAH and propose recommendations for anemia management in SAH patients.

In summary, the studies included in this Special Issue underscore the importance of early recognition of different complication patterns after SAH. The insights gained from these studies may aid in establishing individualized treatment approaches for at-risk patients, thereby improving neurological outcomes. Additionally, in cases involving unruptured CA, precise patient selection for preventive interventions, coupled with efforts to improve intra-procedural safety and ensure the long-term sustainability of treatment outcomes, is imperative. These measures are vital in light of increasing life expectancy. Further research is warranted to corroborate the findings reported in this Special Issue.

Funding: This research received no external funding.

Conflicts of Interest: The authors declare no conflict of interest.

List of Contributions

1. Wach, J.; Vychopen, M.; Güresir, A.; Güresir, E. Anti-Inflammatory Drug Therapy in Aneurysmal Subarachnoid Hemorrhage: A Systematic Review and Meta-Analysis of Prospective Randomized and Placebo-Controlled Trials. *J. Clin. Med.* **2023**, *12*, 4165. https://doi.org/10.3390/jcm12124165.
2. Wójtowicz, K.; Przepiorka, L.; Kujawski, S.; Marchel, A.; Kunert, P. Unruptured Anterior Communicating Artery Aneurysms: Management Strategy and Results of a Single-Center Experience. *J. Clin. Med.* **2023**, *12*, 4619. https://doi.org/10.3390/jcm12144619.
3. Wójtowicz, K.; Przepiorka, L.; Kujawski, S.; Maj, E.; Marchel, A.; Kunert, P. Retrospective Application of Risk Scores to Unruptured Anterior Communicating Artery Aneurysms. *J. Clin. Med.* **2024**, *13*, 789. https://doi.org/10.3390/jcm13030789.
4. Schüngel, M.-S.; Hoffmann, K.-T.; Weber, E.; Maybaum, J.; Bailis, N.; Scheer, M.; Nestler, U.; Schob, S. Distal Flow Diversion with Anti-Thrombotically Coated and Bare Metal Low-Profile Flow Diverters—A Comparison. *J. Clin. Med.* **2023**, *12*, 2700. https://doi.org/10.3390/jcm12072700.

5. Alsbrook, D.L.; Di Napoli, M.; Bhatia, K.; Desai, M.; Hinduja, A.; Rubinos, C.A.; Mansueto, G.; Singh, P.; Domeniconi, G.G.; Ikram, A.; et al. Pathophysiology of Early Brain Injury and Its Association with Delayed Cerebral Ischemia in Aneurysmal Subarachnoid Hemorrhage: A Review of Current Literature. *J. Clin. Med.* **2023**, *12*, 1015. https://doi.org/10.3390/jcm12031015.
6. Said, M.; Gümüs, M.; Rodemerk, J.; Chihi, M.; Rauschenbach, L.; Dinger, T.F.; Oppong, M.D.; Ahmadipour, Y.; Dammann, P.; Wrede, K.H.; et al. Morphometric Study of the Initial Ventricular Indices to Predict the Complications and Outcome of Aneurysmal Subarachnoid Hemorrhage. *J. Clin. Med.* **2023**, *12*, 2585. https://doi.org/10.3390/jcm12072585.
7. Veldeman, M.; Rossmann, T.; Weiss, M.; Conzen-Dilger, C.; Korja, M.; Hoellig, A.; Virta, J.J.; Satopää, J.; Luostarinen, T.; Clusmann, H.; et al. Aneurysmal Subarachnoid Hemorrhage in Hospitalized Patients on Anticoagulants—A Two Center Matched Case-Control Study. *J. Clin. Med.* **2023**, *12*, 1476. https://doi.org/10.3390/jcm12041476.
8. Güresir, E.; Welchowski, T.; Lampmann, T.; Brandecker, S.; Güresir, A.; Wach, J.; Lehmann, F.; Dorn, F.; Velten, M.; Vatter, H. Delayed Cerebral Ischemia after Aneurysmal Subarachnoid Hemorrhage: The Results of Induced Hypertension Only after the IMCVS Trial—A Prospective Cohort Study. *J. Clin. Med.* **2022**, *11*, 5850. https://doi.org/10.3390/jcm11195850.
9. Vatter, H.; Güresir, E.; König, R.; Durner, G.; Kalff, R.; Schuss, P.; Mayer, T.E.; Konczalla, J.; Hattingen, E.; Seifert, V.; et al. Invasive Diagnostic and Therapeutic Management of Cerebral Vasospasm after Aneurysmal Subarachnoid Hemorrhage (IMCVS)—A Phase 2 Randomized Controlled Trial. *J. Clin. Med.* **2022**, *11*, 6197. https://doi.org/10.3390/jcm11206197.
10. Said, M.; Dinger, T.F.; Gümüs, M.; Rauschenbach, L.; Chihi, M.; Rodemerk, J.; Lenz, V.; Oppong, M.D.; Uerschels, A.-K.; Dammann, P.; et al. Impact of Anemia Severity on the Outcome of an Aneurysmal Subarachnoid Hemorrhage. *J. Clin. Med.* **2022**, *11*, 6258. https://doi.org/10.3390/jcm11216258.

References

1. Jabbarli, R.; Rauschenbach, L.; Dinger, T.F.; Darkwah Oppong, M.; Rodemerk, J.; Pierscianek, D.; Dammann, P.; Junker, A.; Sure, U.; Wrede, K.H. In the wall lies the truth: A systematic review of diagnostic markers in intracranial aneurysms. *Brain Pathol.* **2020**, *30*, 437–445. [CrossRef] [PubMed]
2. Vlak, M.H.; Algra, A.; Brandenburg, R.; Rinkel, G.J. Prevalence of unruptured intracranial aneurysms, with emphasis on sex, age, comorbidity, country, and time period: A systematic review and meta-analysis. *Lancet Neurol.* **2011**, *10*, 626–636. [CrossRef] [PubMed]
3. Dinger, T.F.; Peschke, J.; Chihi, M.; Gumus, M.; Said, M.; Santos, A.N.; Rodemerk, J.; Michel, A.; Darkwah Oppong, M.; Li, Y.; et al. Small intracranial aneurysms of the anterior circulation: A negligible risk? *Eur. J. Neurol. Off. J. Eur. Fed. Neurol. Soc.* **2023**, *30*, 389–398. [CrossRef] [PubMed]
4. Darkwah Oppong, M.; Buffen, K.; Pierscianek, D.; Herten, A.; Ahmadipour, Y.; Dammann, P.; Rauschenbach, L.; Forsting, M.; Sure, U.; Jabbarli, R. Secondary hemorrhagic complications in aneurysmal subarachnoid hemorrhage: When the impact hits hard. *J. Neurosurg.* **2019**, 1–8, Online ahead of print. [CrossRef] [PubMed]
5. Jabbarli, R.; Reinhard, M.; Niesen, W.D.; Roelz, R.; Shah, M.; Kaier, K.; Hippchen, B.; Taschner, C.; Van Velthoven, V. Predictors and impact of early cerebral infarction after aneurysmal subarachnoid hemorrhage. *Eur. J. Neurol. Off. J. Eur. Fed. Neurol. Soc.* **2015**, *22*, 941–947. [CrossRef] [PubMed]
6. Lenkeit, A.; Oppong, M.D.; Dinger, T.F.; Gumus, M.; Rauschenbach, L.; Chihi, M.; Ahmadipour, Y.; Uerschels, A.K.; Dammann, P.; Deuschl, C.; et al. Risk factors for poor outcome after aneurysmal subarachnoid hemorrhage in patients with initial favorable neurological status. *Acta Neurochir.* **2024**, *166*, 93. [CrossRef] [PubMed]
7. Said, M.; Gumus, M.; Herten, A.; Dinger, T.F.; Chihi, M.; Darkwah Oppong, M.; Deuschl, C.; Wrede, K.H.; Kleinschnitz, C.; Sure, U.; et al. Subarachnoid Hemorrhage Early Brain Edema Score (SEBES) as a radiographic marker of clinically relevant intracranial hypertension and unfavorable outcome after subarachnoid hemorrhage. *Eur. J. Neurol. Off. J. Eur. Fed. Neurol. Soc.* **2021**, *28*, 4051–4059. [CrossRef]
8. Guresir, E.; Lampmann, T.; Bele, S.; Czabanka, M.; Czorlich, P.; Gempt, J.; Goldbrunner, R.; Hurth, H.; Hermann, E.; Jabbarli, R.; et al. Fight INflammation to Improve outcome after aneurysmal Subarachnoid HEmorRhage (FINISHER) trial: Study protocol for a randomized controlled trial. *Int. J. Stroke Off. J. Int. Stroke Soc.* **2023**, *18*, 242–247. [CrossRef] [PubMed]
9. Dammann, P.; Wittek, P.; Darkwah Oppong, M.; Hutter, B.O.; Jabbarli, R.; Wrede, K.; Wanke, I.; Monninghoff, C.; Kaier, K.; Frank, B.; et al. Relative health-related quality of life after treatment of unruptured intracranial aneurysms: Long-term outcomes and influencing factors. *Ther. Adv. Neurol. Disord.* **2019**, *12*, 1756286419833492. [CrossRef] [PubMed]
10. Jabbarli, R.; Wrede, K.H.; Pierscianek, D.; Dammann, P.; El Hindy, N.; Ozkan, N.; Muller, O.; Stolke, D.; Forsting, M.; Sure, U. Outcome After Clipping of Unruptured Intracranial Aneurysms Depends on Caseload. *World Neurosurg.* **2016**, *89*, 666–671. [CrossRef] [PubMed]

11. Bijlenga, P.; Gondar, R.; Schilling, S.; Morel, S.; Hirsch, S.; Cuony, J.; Corniola, M.V.; Perren, F.; Rufenacht, D.; Schaller, K. PHASES Score for the Management of Intracranial Aneurysm: A Cross-Sectional Population-Based Retrospective Study. *Stroke* **2017**, *48*, 2105–2112. [CrossRef] [PubMed]
12. Etminan, N.; Brown, R.D., Jr.; Beseoglu, K.; Juvela, S.; Raymond, J.; Morita, A.; Torner, J.C.; Derdeyn, C.P.; Raabe, A.; Mocco, J.; et al. The unruptured intracranial aneurysm treatment score: A multidisciplinary consensus. *Neurology* **2015**, *85*, 881–889. [CrossRef] [PubMed]
13. Greving, J.P.; Wermer, M.J.; Brown, R.D., Jr.; Morita, A.; Juvela, S.; Yonekura, M.; Ishibashi, T.; Torner, J.C.; Nakayama, T.; Rinkel, G.J.; et al. Development of the PHASES score for prediction of risk of rupture of intracranial aneurysms: A pooled analysis of six prospective cohort studies. *Lancet Neurol.* **2014**, *13*, 59–66. [CrossRef] [PubMed]
14. Opitz, M.; Zenk, C.; Zensen, S.; Bos, D.; Li, Y.; Styczen, H.; Oppong, M.D.; Jabbarli, R.; Hagenacker, T.; Forsting, M.; et al. Radiation dose and fluoroscopy time of aneurysm coiling in patients with unruptured and ruptured intracranial aneurysms as a function of aneurysm size, location, and patient age. *Neuroradiology* **2023**, *65*, 637–644. [CrossRef] [PubMed]
15. Fatania, K.; Patankar, D.T. Comprehensive review of the recent advances in devices for endovascular treatment of complex brain aneurysms. *Br. J. Radiol.* **2022**, *95*, 20210538. [CrossRef] [PubMed]
16. Said, M.; Gumus, M.; Rodemerk, J.; Chihi, M.; Rauschenbach, L.; Dinger, T.F.; Darkwah Oppong, M.; Dammann, P.; Wrede, K.H.; Sure, U.; et al. The value of ventricular measurements in the prediction of shunt dependency after aneurysmal subarachnoid hemorrhage. *Acta Neurochir.* **2023**, *165*, 1545–1555. [CrossRef] [PubMed]
17. Said, M.; Gumus, M.; Rodemerk, J.; Rauschenbach, L.; Chihi, M.; Dinger, T.F.; Darkwah Oppong, M.; Schmidt, B.; Ahmadipour, Y.; Dammann, P.; et al. Systematic review and meta-analysis of outcome-relevant anemia in patients with subarachnoid hemorrhage. *Sci. Rep.* **2022**, *12*, 20738. [CrossRef] [PubMed]

Disclaimer/Publisher's Note: The statements, opinions and data contained in all publications are solely those of the individual author(s) and contributor(s) and not of MDPI and/or the editor(s). MDPI and/or the editor(s) disclaim responsibility for any injury to people or property resulting from any ideas, methods, instructions or products referred to in the content.

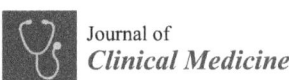

Journal of *Clinical Medicine*

Article

Invasive Diagnostic and Therapeutic Management of Cerebral VasoSpasm after Aneurysmal Subarachnoid Hemorrhage (IMCVS)—A Phase 2 Randomized Controlled Trial

Hartmut Vatter [1,*,†], Erdem Güresir [1,†], Ralph König [2], Gregor Durner [2], Rolf Kalff [3], Patrick Schuss [1], Thomas E. Mayer [4], Jürgen Konczalla [5], Elke Hattingen [6], Volker Seifert [5] and Joachim Berkefeld [6]

1. Department of Neurosurgery, University Hospital Bonn, 53127 Bonn, Germany
2. Department of Neurosurgery, University of Ulm, Günzburg, 89081 Ulm, Germany
3. Department of Neurosurgery, Jena University Hospital, 07743 Jena, Germany
4. Department of Neuroradiology, Jena University Hospital, 07743 Jena, Germany
5. Department of Neurosurgery, University Hospital Frankfurt, 60590 Frankfurt am Main, Germany
6. Department of Neuroradiology, University Hospital Frankfurt, 60590 Frankfurt am Main, Germany
* Correspondence: hartmut.vatter@ukbonn.de; Tel.: +49-228-287-16521
† These authors contributed equally to this work.

Abstract: Cerebral vasospasm (CVS) is associated with delayed cerebral ischemia (DCI) after aneurysmal subarachnoid hemorrhage (SAH). The most frequently used form of rescue therapy for CVS is invasive endovascular therapy. Due to a lack of prospective data, we performed a prospective randomized multicenter trial (NCT01400360). A total of 34 patients in three centers were randomized to invasive endovascular treatment or conservative therapy at diagnosis of relevant CVS onset. Imaging data was assessed by a neuroradiologist blinded for treatment allocation. Primary outcome measure was development of DCI. Secondary endpoints included clinical outcome at 6 months after SAH. A total of 18 of the 34 patients were treated conservatively, and 16 patients were treated with invasive endovascular treatment for CVS. There was no statistical difference in the rate of cerebral infarctions either at initial or at the follow-up MRI between the groups. However, the outcome at 6 months was better in patients treated conservatively (mRs 2 ± 1.5 vs. 4 ± 1.8, $p = 0.005$). Invasive endovascular treatment for CVS does not lead to a lower rate of DCI but might lead to poorer outcomes compared to induced hypertension. The potential benefits of endovascular treatment for CVS need to be addressed in further studies, searching for a subgroup of patients who may benefit.

Keywords: intracranial aneurysm; treatment; subarachnoid hemorrhage; vasospasm; delayed ischemic neurological deficit; balloon angioplasty; intra-arterial spasmolysis

1. Introduction

Delayed cerebral ischemia (DCI) is an important cause of poor outcome after an aneurysmal subarachnoid hemorrhage (SAH) and is defined as a focal neurological impairment or a decrease of the patients' Glasgow coma scale score as defined by Vergouwen et al [1,2]. Currently, orally administered Nimodipine is the only intervention to prevent DCI after SAH. However, this effect of Nimodipine seems to be due to neuroprotection rather than by vasodilation [3]. Cerebral vasospasm (CVS) is associated with DCI [4] that may develop by lowering cerebral blood supply below demand.

At present, medical therapy for CVS is induced hypertension [5]. The most frequently used form of rescue therapy for CVS is invasive endovascular therapy, including selective intra-arterial infusion of vasodilators and balloon angioplasty [6,7]. Due to a lack of prospective data for invasive diagnostic and the therapeutic management of CVS, we performed a prospective randomized study comparing DCI-related infarctions and the clinical outcome of patients with SAH and CVS with and without invasive endovascular treatment (NCT01400360).

2. Materials and Methods

Between August 2009 and September 2012, we performed a multicenter, randomized trial in 3 hospitals in Germany (University Hospital Frankfurt, University Hospital Ulm, and University Hospital Jena). The study was approved by the local ethics committee and all participating centers (Ethik-Kommission, University Hospital Frankfurt, ID 68/09). Written informed consent was obtained from all patients.

2.1. Definitions and Data Recording

SAH was diagnosed by computed tomography (CT) or lumbar puncture. All patients with spontaneous SAH underwent four-vessel digital subtraction angiography (DSA). Clinical data, including patient characteristics on admission and during treatment course, radiological features, and functional neurological outcome were collected and entered into a computerized database (SPSS Version 15 Institute, Inc, Chicago, IL, USA). Treatment decision (coiling versus clipping) was based on an interdisciplinary approach in each individual case. Aneurysm treatment was performed within 24 h after admission. Acute hydrocephalus was treated by external cerebrospinal fluid diversion. Osmotherapy and mild hyperventilation were used for the treatment of elevated ICP (>20 mmHg). Apart from close neurological monitoring, routine surveillance included daily transcranial Doppler measurements of red blood cell flow velocities. CT imaging was performed routinely (1) 24–48 h after aneurysm clip or coil obliteration to assess procedural complications, (2) on day 14–21 to diagnose delayed cerebral infarctions and to assess the necessity of a ventriculoperitoneal shunt, and (3) at variable time points whenever neurological deteriorations occurred. All patients underwent screening for CVS using MRI, including PWI/DWI, performed routinely on day 4–14 and cerebral angiography between day 7 and 10 [7]. Baseline MRI with PWI/DWI was also performed in any case of neurological deterioration of the patient or increased mean velocity $\geq$150 cm/s or an increase in velocity $\geq$50 cm/s within 24 h in transcranial Doppler sonography. Sufficient fluid was administered to maintain a high normal euvolemic status. All patients received nimodipine from the day of admission. In the case of hyponatremia fludrocortisone was added to the therapy.

2.2. Inclusion Criteria

Patient age of 18–75 years. Patients who could undergo MRI scans initially and at follow-up. Patients with aneurysmal SAH WFNS grades I–IV with hemodynamically relevant CVS defined as: 1. Elevated time to peak (TTP) > 2 s compared to the corresponding contralateral side, or mean transit time (MTT) > 3.5 s. 2. Profound narrowing of cerebral vessels in MRA scan. 3. Existence of "tissue at risk" (vital brain tissue with DWI lesions <50%), as described before [8].

Patients were then randomized in one of the two groups, conservative versus invasive endovascular treatment, in a 1:1 allocation ratio. Patients without relevant CVS in DSA, patients with DWI lesions $\geq$ 50% of the relevant vessel territory, and patients who were not able to undergo MRI scans due to moribund clinical status or due to implants not safe for MRI imaging, as well as patients WFNS grade V, were excluded from the study.

2.3. Randomization

Patients were then randomized in one of the two groups, conservative versus invasive endovascular treatment, in a 1:1 allocation ratio (Figure 1). Patients without relevant CVS in DSA, patients with DWI lesions $\geq$ 50% of the relevant vessel territory, and patients who were not able to undergo MRI scans due to moribund clinical status or due to implants not safe for MRI imaging, as well as patients WFNS grade V, were excluded from the study.

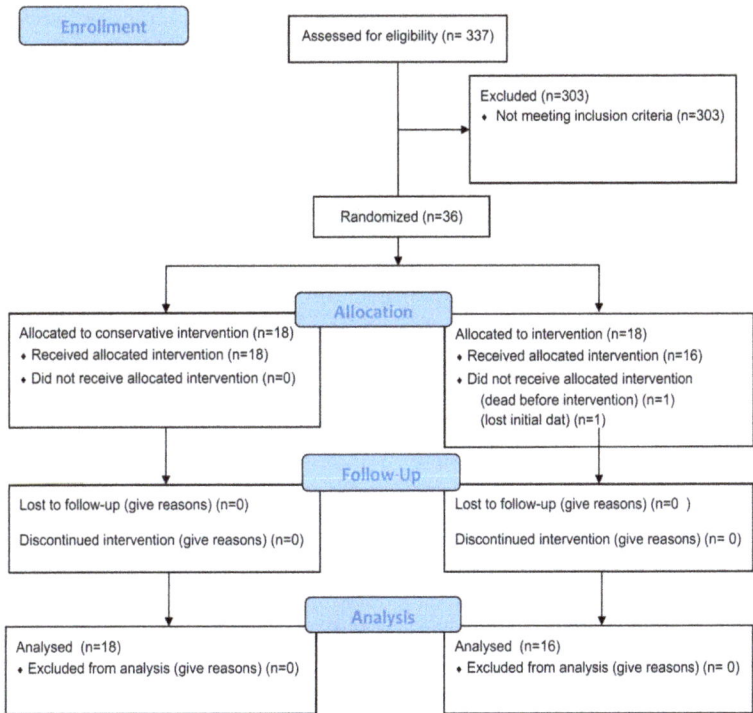

Figure 1. Diagram illustrating the flowchart regarding assessment, randomization, allocation, follow-up, and final analysis of study patients.

2.4. Conservative Treatment

Arterial hypertension was induced with norepinephrine and fluids via central venous line. Mean arterial blood pressure (MAP) was raised to 110 mmHg. Induced hypertension was continued for 7 days. Thereafter, patients were reassessed for CVS using MRI. In patients with CVS, induced hypertension was continued for the following 7 days, and reassessment was performed thereafter, as described above. In patients with resolution of CVS, induced hypertension was terminated.

2.5. Invasive Endovascular Treatment

Whenever possible, proximal CVS was treated by transluminal balloon angioplasty (TBA) and distal or diffuse CVS was treated by intra-arterial application of nimodipine at the discretion of the treating neuroradiologist, as described previously [9,10].

2.6. Outcome Measurement and Endpoints

The flowchart of the diagnosis and treatment protocol, as well as the efficacy assessment of endovascular therapy, is published in Vatter et al. 2011 [8]. Efficacy of endovascular treatment was assessed by the treating neuroradiologist and graded into good versus fair. The effect of endovascular treatment was controlled 48 ± 12 h later with MRI. In case of DWI/PWI mismatch, the treatment cycle consisting of MRI, DSA (including endovascular treatment), and a follow-up MRI (48 ± 12 h later) was repeated until no further tissue at risk could be detected.

Imaging data for new infarctions during the phase of CVS was assessed by a neuroradiologist blinded for treatment allocation. The cerebrum was partitioned into 19 segments. A 50% DWI lesion ≥ 1 segment was defined as major and < 50% was defined as minor infarct. Only delayed spontaneous infarctions were counted as DCI-related cerebral infarctions.

Lesions related to aneurysm treatment (clipping or coiling of the ruptured aneurysm) or caused by extraventricular drains, pre-existing infarcts, and hypodensities surrounding hematoma or in proximity to the site of surgery were excluded.

The primary outcome measure was the development of new DCI-related cerebral infarctions during the phase of CVS. Secondary endpoints included clinical outcome at 6 months after SAH according to the modified Rankin scale (mRs).

2.7. Sample Size Calculation

As 60–75% of SAH patients with relevant CVS ("tissue at risk") develop DCI [11–13], the study was planned to decrease CVS related infarcts to 50% by invasive endovascular diagnostic and management, with $\alpha = 0.05$, and 80% power, for which 92 patients in a 1:1 randomization was needed. An interim analysis was planned after 34 patients.

2.8. Statistics

Data analyses were performed using the computer software package SPSS (IBM SPSS Statistics for Windows, Version 25.0. IBM Corp., Armonk, NY, USA). Unpaired t-test was used for parametric statistics. Categorical variables were analyzed in contingency tables using Fisher's exact test. Results with $p < 0.05$ were considered statistically significant.

3. Results

3.1. Patient Characteristics

A total of 34 patients had CVS. Eighteen patients were treated conservatively, and sixteen patients were treated with invasive endovascular treatment for CVS (Table 1).

Table 1. Patient characteristics.

Variable	Conservative (n = 18)	Invasive (n = 16)	p-Value
Age, Y ± SD, mean	55 ± 10	56 ± 12	
Smoker	9/14	9/14	1.0
Diabetes	0/18	2/15	0.2
Hypertension before SAH	8/18	8/15	0.7
Coronary heart disease	2/18	0/16	0.5
Adipositas	1/12	1/15	1.0
BMI	27 ± 3	22 ± 0.4	0.4
History of malignoma	0	0	
History of cerebral ischemia	1/18	1/16	
Extensive alcohol consumption	2/18	1/16	
History of myocardial infarction	2/18	0	
History of SAH (from the same aneurysm)	1/18	0	
mRS before SAH	0	0	
Karnofsky before SAH	100 ± 0	99 ± 3	0.1
Hydrocephalus at admission	13/16	12/16	1.0
GCS	9 ± 5	8 ± 4	0.6
WFNS grade	4 ± 2	4 ± 1	0.6
Fisher score	3 ± 0.5	3 ± 0.4	0.2
IVH	5/16	4/14	1.0
ICH < 3 cm	2/15	5/15	0.1
ICH > 3 cm	2/15	5/15	0.1
Clipping	10/18	8/18 *	
Coiling	8/18	10/18 *	

* number of patients assigned to invasive treatment. BMI = body mass index; GCS = Glasgow coma scale; ICH = intracerebral hemorrhage; IVH = intraventricular hemorrhage; mRS = modified Rankin scale; SAH = subarachnoid hemorrhage; Y = years.

3.2. Initial MRI

Of the 18 patients treated conservatively, 5 patients had no DWI lesions, 10 patients had minor DWI lesions, and 3 patients had major DWI lesions in the initial MRI.

Of the 16 patients in the invasive endovascular group, 2 patients had no DWI lesions, 11 patients had minor DWI lesions, and 3 patients had major DWI lesions in the initial MRI.

The initial rate of no/minor DWI lesions compared to major DWI lesions did not differ between the assigned treatment groups ($p = 1.0$).

3.3. Follow-Up MRI

Of the 18 patients treated conservatively, 8 patients had no new DWI lesion, 7 patients had new minor DWI lesions, and 3 patients had major DWI lesions in the follow-up MRI.

Of the 16 patients in the invasive endovascular treatment group, 8 patients had no new DWI lesion, 4 patients had new minor DWI lesions, and 4 patients had major DWI lesions in the follow-up MRI.

The rate of no new/new minor DWI lesions compared to new major DWI lesions did not differ between the assigned treatment groups ($p = 0.7$).

3.4. Frequency, Success, and Complications of Endovascular Treatment

Of the 16 patients who underwent invasive endovascular treatment, 16 patients underwent one procedure, 11 patients underwent two procedures, 4 patients underwent three procedures, 2 patients underwent four procedures, and one patient underwent five procedures. Detailed data on frequency, success, and complications of invasive endovascular treatment are presented in Tables 2 and 3.

Table 2. Invasive endovascular treatment.

Frequency of DSA	No. of pts.	Endovascular Treatment (i.a. Nimodipine/PTA)	No. of pts.	Treatment Success According to Interventionalist
1	16	i.a. nimodipine	16	Good (16/16)
2	11	i.a. nimodipine	7/11	Good (4/10)
				Fair (3/10)
		PTA	3/11	Good (3/10)
		none	1/11	Massive thromboembolic event
3	4	i.a. nimodipine	3/4	Good (1/4)
				Fair (1/4)
				No success (1/4)
		PTA	1/4	Good (1/4)
4	2	i.a. nimodipine	2	Good (0/2)
				Fair (1/2)
				No success (1/2)
5	1	i.a. nimodipine	1	Fair (1/1)

Table 3. Complications of invasive endovascular treatment.

Frequency of DSA	No. of pts.	Complications	No. of pts.	Severity of Complication/Necessity of Treatment
1	16	None		
2	11	Dissection	1	Stent implantation
		Bleeding	0	
		Thromboembolic event	1	Minor supratentorial infarction
		Embolic infarction	1	Massive cerebellar and brainstem infarction
3	4	Dissection	1	Stent implantation
		Bleeding	0	
		Thromboembolic event	1	Major supratentorial infarction
		Embolic infarction	0	
4	2	Dissection	0	
		Bleeding	0	
		Thromboembolic event	0	
		Embolic infarction	0	
5	1	None		

3.5. Outcome

Clinical outcome after 6 months was better in patients treated conservatively compared to patients in the invasive endovascular treatment group (mRs 2 ± 1.5 vs. 4 ± 1.8, $p = 0.004$, Figure 2).

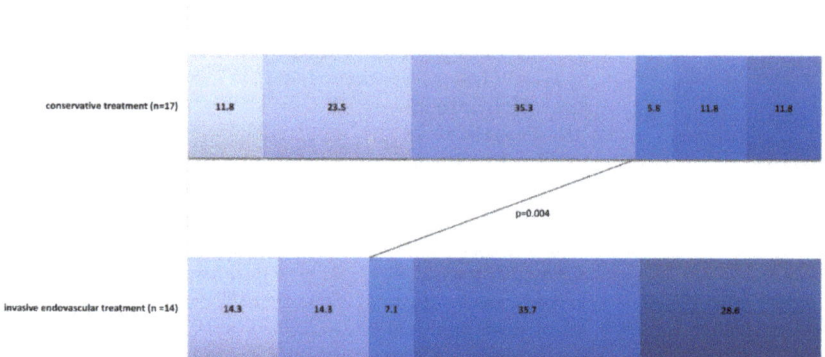

Figure 2. Column bars showing the proportions of patients regarding the mRS after 6 months. The first column bar represents the conservative treatment arm, whereas the second bar displays the invasive endovascular treatment arm. The line connects the mean mRS values of both groups and the *p*-value represents the result of the independent *t*-test.

4. Discussion

In this randomized trial, patients in the conservative treatment group, i.e., treatment with induced hypertension after diagnosis of CVS, had a better clinical outcome compared to patients in the invasive endovascular group. Therefore, the study was stopped prematurely after randomization of 34 patients.

Induced hypertension with maintenance of euvolemia is currently used in order to perform hemodynamic augmentation [14] and increase cerebral blood flow as well as brain tissue oxygenation [15].

Suwatcharangkoon et al. [16] recently showed that failure to respond to induced hypertension in patients with symptomatic vasospasm leads to a higher rate of cerebral infarction and poor outcome after 1 year compared to the group of patients who respond to induced hypertension.

According to the guidelines for the management of SAH [14], induced hypertension is recommended in patients with symptomatic CVS. While the prematurely terminated study on Hypertension Induction in the Management of AneurysmaL subarachnoid haemorrhage with secondary IschaemiA (HIMALAIA) [17] did not support induced hypertension, it was underpowered to draw definitive conclusions. In a retrospective observational study, Haegens et al. [18] analyzed SAH patients with diagnosed CVS and compared DCI rates in the group of patients with induced hypertension and without. DCI rates were significantly lower in the induced hypertension group (20%) compared to the group without induced hypertension (33%). Furthermore, Haegens et al. concluded that the reduced DCI rates may also lead to a reduction of poor clinical outcome.

Patients with CVS at the ICU reflect a highly vulnerable subgroup of SAH patients who are at risk for DCI that may develop when cerebral blood supply decreases below demand. An invasive diagnostic and therapeutic management in patients with critically low cerebral blood supply may lead to varying blood pressure and decreased monitoring compared to the treatment at the ICU over a period of time, which may explain why the otherwise effective treatment of angiographic CVS does not translate into better outcomes [19].

Furthermore, CVS is only one explanation for poor outcome after SAH. It is possible that factors such as early brain injury or systemic illness may contribute to poor outcome.

In conclusion, invasive endovascular treatment seems to be effective in the treatment of visual CVS. However, despite its widespread use nowadays, there is no evidence that invasive endovascular treatment improves outcome in patients with CVS, whereas it seems to have a high rate of serious complications [20]. A possible benefit of invasive endovascular treatment on clinical outcome could be limited to a special subgroup of SAH patients with CVS; however, it is unclear which patient cohort this subgroup might be.

We therefore changed our treatment policy in patients with diagnosed CVS to induced hypertension only and published our prospective results in the subgroup of SAH patients meeting inclusion criteria of the IMCVS trial recently [21].

Limitations

The most obvious limitation is the limited power due to the smaller study population size than planned. Therefore, the potential benefits of invasive diagnostic and endovascular treatment cannot be ruled out. However, the randomized controlled design and a clear definition of CVS are the strengths of the trial. Furthermore, the result that clinical outcome of patients in the group of invasive diagnostic and therapeutic management compared to the conservative group is not only similar, but significantly poorer, does not support the widespread use of endovascular treatment for CVS but necessitates further studies in order define a subgroup of SAH patients who may benefit from this kind of invasive treatment.

5. Conclusions

In conclusion, we found that invasive endovascular treatment in SAH patients with CVS does not lead to a lower rate of delayed cerebral ischemia or improved clinical outcome but might lead to poorer outcome compared to patients treated with induced hypertension for CVS. Potential benefits of endovascular treatment for CVS need to be addressed in further studies, searching for a subgroup of patients who may benefit.

Author Contributions: Conceptualization, E.G., J.B. and H.V.; methodology, E.G., H.V. and J.B.; data curation, H.V., E.G., R.K. (Ralph König), G.D., R.K. (Rolf Kalff), T.E.M., J.K., E.H., V.S. and J.B.; writing—original draft preparation, H.V., E.G. and J.B.; writing—review and editing, H.V., E.G., R.K. (Ralph König), G.D., R.K. (Rolf Kalff), P.S., T.E.M., J.K., E.H., V.S., J.B. and E.G.; visualization, E.G.; supervision, E.G. and H.V. All authors have read and agreed to the published version of the manuscript.

Funding: This research received no external funding.

Institutional Review Board Statement: The study was conducted according to the guidelines of the Declaration of Helsinki and approved by the Ethics Committee of the Medical Faculty and the University Hospital of Frankfurt (code: 68/09).

Informed Consent Statement: Written informed consent was obtained from all patients.

Data Availability Statement: All data are included in this manuscript.

Conflicts of Interest: The authors declare no conflict of interest.

References

1. Vergouwen, M.D.; Vermeulen, M.; van Gijn, J.; Rinkel, G.J.; Wijdicks, E.F.; Muizelaar, J.P.; Mendelow, A.D.; Juvela, S.; Yonas, H.; Terbrugge, K.G.; et al. Definition of delayed cerebral ischemia after aneurysmal subarachnoid hemorrhage as an outcome event in clinical trials and observational studies: Proposal of a multidisciplinary research group. *Stroke* **2010**, *41*, 2391–2395. [CrossRef] [PubMed]
2. Roos, Y.B.; de Haan, R.J.; Beenen, L.F.; Groen, R.J.; Albrecht, K.W.; Vermeulen, M. Complications and outcome in patients with aneurysmal subarachnoid haemorrhage: A prospective hospital based cohort study in the Netherlands. *J. Neurol. Neurosurg. Psychiatry* **2000**, *68*, 337–341. [CrossRef] [PubMed]
3. Mees, S.D.; Rinkel, G.J.; Feigin, V.L.; Algra, A.; Bergh, W.M.V.D.; Vermeulen, M.; Van Gijn, J. Calcium antagonists for aneurysmal subarachnoid haemorrhage. *Cochrane Database Syst. Rev.* **2007**, *2007*, CD000277.

4. Schmidt, J.M.; Wartenberg, K.E.; Fernandez, A.; Claassen, J.; Rincon, F.; Ostapkovich, N.D.; Badjatia, N.; Parra, A.; Connolly, E.S.; Mayer, S.A. Frequency and clinical impact of asymptomatic cerebral infarction due to vasospasm after subarachnoid hemorrhage. *J. Neurosurg.* **2008**, *109*, 1052–1059. [CrossRef] [PubMed]
5. Muizelaar, J.P.; Becker, D.P. Induced hypertension for the treatment of cerebral ischemia after subarachnoid hemorrhage. Direct effect on cerebral blood flow. *Surg. Neurol.* **1986**, *25*, 317–325. [CrossRef]
6. Bulsara, K.R.; Gunel, M.; Amin-Hanjani, S.; Chen, P.R.; Connolly, E.S.; Friedlander, R.M. Results of a national cerebrovascular neurosurgery survey on the management of cerebral vasospasm/delayed cerebral ischemia. *J. Neurointerv. Surg.* **2015**, *7*, 408–411. [CrossRef]
7. Boulouis, G.; Labeyrie, M.A.; Raymond, J.; Rodriguez-Régent, C.; Lukaszewicz, A.C.; Bresson, D.; Ben Hassen, W.; Trystram, D.; Meder, J.F.; Oppenheim, C.; et al. Treatment of cerebral vasospasm following aneurysmal subarachnoid haemorrhage: A systematic review and meta-analysis. *Eur. Radiol.* **2017**, *27*, 3333–3342. [CrossRef]
8. Vatter, H.; Güresir, E.; Berkefeld, J.; Beck, J.; Raabe, A.; Rochemont, R.D.M.D.; Seifert, V.; Weidauer, S. Perfusion-diffusion mismatch in MRI to indicate endovascular treatment of cerebral vasospasm after subarachnoid haemorrhage. *J. Neurol. Neurosurg. Psychiatry* **2011**, *82*, 876–883. [CrossRef]
9. Beck, J.; Raabe, A.; Lanfermann, H.; Berkefeld, J.; Rochemont, R.D.M.D.; Zanella, F.; Seifert, V.; Weidauer, S. Effects of balloon angioplasty on perfusion- and diffusion-weighted magnetic resonance imaging results and outcome in patients with cerebral vasospasm. *J. Neurosurg.* **2006**, *105*, 220–227. [CrossRef]
10. Turowski, B.; du Mesnil de Rochemont, R.; Beck, J.; Berkefeld, J.; Zanella, F.E. Assessment of changes in cerebral circulation time due to vasospasm in a specific arterial territory: Effect of angioplasty. *Neuroradiology* **2005**, *47*, 134–143. [CrossRef] [PubMed]
11. Beck, J.; Raabe, A.; Lanfermann, H.; Seifert, V.; Weidauer, S. Tissue at risk concept for endovascular treatment of severe vasospasm after aneurysmal subarachnoid haemorrhage. *J. Neurol. Neurosurg. Psychiatry* **2004**, *75*, 1779–1781. [CrossRef] [PubMed]
12. Weidauer, S.; Lanfermann, H.; Raabe, A.; Zanella, F.; Seifert, V.; Beck, J. Impairment of cerebral perfusion and infarct patterns attributable to vasospasm after aneurysmal subarachnoid hemorrhage: A prospective MRI and DSA study. *Stroke* **2007**, *38*, 1831–1836. [CrossRef] [PubMed]
13. Weidauer, S.; Vatter, H.; Beck, J.; Raabe, A.; Lanfermann, H.; Seifert, V.; Zanella, F. Focal laminar cortical infarcts following aneurysmal subarachnoid haemorrhage. *Neuroradiology* **2008**, *50*, 1–8. [CrossRef]
14. Connolly, E.S., Jr.; Rabinstein, A.A.; Carhuapoma, J.R.; Derdeyn, C.P.; Dion, J.; Higashida, R.T.; Hoh, B.L.; Kirkness, C.J.; Naidech, A.M.; Ogilvy, C.S.; et al. Guidelines for the management of aneurysmal subarachnoid hemorrhage: A guideline for healthcare professionals from the American Heart Association/american Stroke Association. *Stroke* **2012**, *43*, 1711–1737. [CrossRef] [PubMed]
15. Muench, E.; Horn, P.; Bauhuf, C.; Roth, H.; Philipps, M.; Hermann, P.; Quintel, M.; Schmiedek, P.; Vajkoczy, P. Effects of hypervolemia and hypertension on regional cerebral blood flow, intracranial pressure, and brain tissue oxygenation after subarachnoid hemorrhage. *Crit. Care Med.* **2007**, *35*, 1844–1851. [CrossRef] [PubMed]
16. Suwatcharangkoon, S.; De Marchis, G.M.; Witsch, J.; Meyers, E.; Velazquez, A.; Falo, C.; Schmidt, J.M.; Agarwal, S.; Connolly, E.S.; Claassen, J.; et al. Medical Treatment Failure for Symptomatic Vasospasm After Subarachnoid Hemorrhage Threatens Long-Term Outcome. *Stroke* **2019**, *50*, 1696–1702. [CrossRef]
17. Gathier, C.S.; van den Bergh, W.M.; van der Jagt, M.; Verweij, B.H.; Dankbaar, J.W.; Müller, M.C.; Oldenbeuving, A.W.; Rinkel, G.J.; Slooter, A.J. Induced Hypertension for Delayed Cerebral Ischemia After Aneurysmal Subarachnoid Hemorrhage: A Randomized Clinical Trial. *Stroke* **2018**, *49*, 76–83. [CrossRef] [PubMed]
18. Haegens, N.M.; Gathier, C.S.; Horn, J.; Coert, B.A.; Verbaan, D.; van den Bergh, W.M. Induced Hypertension in Preventing Cerebral Infarction in Delayed Cerebral Ischemia After Subarachnoid Hemorrhage. *Stroke* **2018**, *49*, 2630–2636. [CrossRef]
19. Hosmann, A.; Angelmayr, C.; Hopf, A.; Rauscher, S.; Brugger, J.; Ritscher, L.; Bohl, I.; Schnackenburg, P.; Engel, A.; Plöchl, W.; et al. Detrimental effects of intrahospital transport on cerebral metabolism in patients suffering severe aneurysmal subarachnoid hemorrhage. *J. Neurosurg.* **2021**, 1–8. [CrossRef]
20. Adami, D.; Berkefeld, J.; Platz, J.; Konczalla, J.; Pfeilschifter, W.; Weidauer, S.; Wagner, M. Complication rate of intraarterial treatment of severe cerebral vasospasm after subarachnoid hemorrhage with nimodipine and percutaneous transluminal balloon angioplasty: Worth the risk? *J. Neuroradiol.* **2019**, *46*, 15–24. [CrossRef]
21. Güresir, E.; Welchowski, T.; Lampmann, T.; Brandecker, S.; Güresir, A.; Wach, J.; Lehmann, F.; Dorn, F.; Velten, M.; Vatter, H. Delayed Cerebral Ischemia after Aneurysmal Subarachnoid Hemorrhage: The Results of Induced Hypertension Only after the IMCVS Trial—A Prospective Cohort Study. *J. Clin. Med.* **2022**, *11*, 5850. [CrossRef] [PubMed]

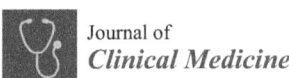

Journal of Clinical Medicine

Article

Delayed Cerebral Ischemia after Aneurysmal Subarachnoid Hemorrhage: The Results of Induced Hypertension Only after the IMCVS Trial—A Prospective Cohort Study

Erdem Güresir [1,*], Thomas Welchowski [2], Tim Lampmann [1], Simon Brandecker [1], Agi Güresir [1], Johannes Wach [1], Felix Lehmann [2], Franziska Dorn [3], Markus Velten [4] and Hartmut Vatter [1]

[1] Department of Neurosurgery, University Hospital Bonn, 53127 Bonn, Germany
[2] Institute of Medical Biometry, Informatics and Epidemiology, University Hospital Bonn, 53127 Bonn, Germany
[3] Department of Neuroradiology, University Hospital Bonn, 53127 Bonn, Germany
[4] Department of Anesthesiology and Intensive Care, University Hospital Bonn, 53127 Bonn, Germany
* Correspondence: erdem.gueresir@ukbonn.de; Tel.: +49-228-287-16521

Abstract: Delayed cerebral ischemia (DCI) is a predictor of poor outcome after aneurysmal subarachnoid hemorrhage (SAH). Treatment strategies vary and include induced hypertension and invasive endovascular treatment. After the IMCVS trial (NCT01400360), which failed to demonstrate a benefit of endovascular treatment for cerebral vasospasm (CVS) and resulted in a significantly worse outcome, we changed our treatment policy in patients with diagnosed CVS to induced hypertension only, and we present our prospective results in the subgroup of SAH patients meeting inclusion criteria of the IMCVS trial. All patients underwent screening for DIND when conscious and for CVS using CT-A/-P at day 6–8 after SAH. In the case of CVS, arterial hypertension was induced and continued until re-assessment. In total, 149 of 303 patients developed CVS. DCI developed in 35 patients (23.5%). In multivariate analyses, CVS was a predictor for the development of new infarctions. Poor admission status, re-bleeding before treatment, and DCI predicted poor outcome. The omittance of invasive endovascular rescue therapies in SAH patients with CVS, additional to induced hypertension, does not lead to a higher rate of DCI. Potential benefits of additional endovascular treatment for CVS need to be addressed in further studies searching for a subgroup of patients who may benefit.

Keywords: intracranial aneurysm; treatment; subarachnoid hemorrhage; vasospasm; delayed ischemic neurological deficit

1. Introduction

Delayed cerebral ischemia (DCI) is associated with cerebral vasospasm (CVS) and is a common cause of poor outcome after aneurysmal subarachnoid hemorrhage (SAH) [1]. To improve outcome, rescue therapies including selective intraarterial infusion of vasodilators, balloon angioplasty, and induced hypertension are used [2]. Due to a lack of prospective data for the invasive diagnostic and therapeutic management of CVS, as well as the considerable inconsistency of its screening, a randomized clinical trial was initiated to assess the influences of a structured assessment of CVS and of rescue therapies on new cerebral infarctions during the phase of CVS and clinical outcome (Invasive diagnostic and therapeutic management of cerebral vasospasm after aneurysmal subarachnoid hemorrhage, IMCVS trial NCT01400360). Patients in the IMCVS trial underwent screening for CVS using MRI, performed routinely on days 4–14, and cerebral angiography between days 7–10. MRI was also performed in any case of neurological deterioration of the patient or increased mean velocity ≥150 cm/s or an increase in velocity ≥50 cm/s within 24 h in transcranial Doppler sonography. Patients with hemodynamically relevant CVS defined as 1. elevated time to peak (TTP) > 2 s compared to the corresponding contralateral side,

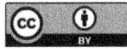

or mean transit time (MTT) > 3.5 s, 2. profound narrowing of cerebral vessels in MRA scan, and 3. existence of "tissue at risk" (vital brain tissue with DWI lesions <50%) were randomized into a conservative group versus invasive endovascular treatment group. Conservative treatment consisted of induced hypertension (mean arterial blood pressure raised to 110 mmHg). Invasive endovascular treatment consisted of transluminal balloon angioplasty (TBA) for proximal CVS whenever possible, and/or intraarterial application of nimodipine for distal or diffuse CVS. The primary outcome measure was the development of new cerebral infarctions. After the IMCVS trial failed to demonstrate a radiological and clinical benefit of endovascular treatment, the trial was stopped prematurely because of safety concerns. In the following, we changed our treatment policy in patients with diagnosed CVS to induced hypertension only and present our prospective results in the subgroup of SAH patients meeting inclusion criteria of the IMCVS trial.

2. Materials and Methods

Between January 2013 and January 2020, 303 patients with SAH (WFNS 1–4), meeting the inclusion criteria of the IMCVS trial, were treated in the authors' institution. The study was approved by the local ethics committee (Ethikkommission, University of Bonn, ID 331/12), waiving patient informed consent for the observational study.

2.1. Definitions and Clinical Workflow

SAH was diagnosed by computed tomography (CT) or lumbar puncture. All patients with spontaneous SAH underwent four-vessel digital subtraction angiography (DSA). Clinical data, including patient characteristics on admission and during treatment course, radiological features, and functional neurological outcome were collected and entered into a computerized database (IBM SPSS Statistics for Windows, Version 25.0. Armonk, NY, USA, IBM Corp.). Treatment decision (coil/clip) was based on an interdisciplinary approach in each individual case. Aneurysm treatment was performed within 24 h after admission. Acute hydrocephalus was treated by external cerebrospinal fluid diversion. Osmotherapy and mild hyperventilation were used for the treatment of elevated ICP (>20 mmHg). Apart from close neurological monitoring, routine surveillance included continuous invasive blood-pressure monitoring using an arterial catheter, daily transcranial Doppler measurements of red blood cell flow velocities, and ICP monitoring, as well as continuous electroencephalography in selected cases. Furthermore, CT-imaging was performed routinely (1) 24–48 h after the aneurysm clip or coil obliteration to assess procedural complications, (2) on day 14–21 to diagnose delayed cerebral infarctions and to assess the necessity of a ventriculoperitoneal shunt, and (3) at variable time points whenever neurological deteriorations occurred. All patients underwent screening for DIND when conscious, and for CVS using CT-A/CT-P at days 6–8 after SAH. In the case of CVS, arterial hypertension was induced as described in detail below and continued until re-assessment 7 days later. Sufficient fluid was administered to maintain a high normal euvolemic status. All patients received nimodipine from the day of admission. In the case of hyponatremia, fludrocortisone was added to the therapy.

2.2. Data recording and Clinical Outcome Measurement

Information, including patient characteristics, treatment modality, aneurysm size and location, radiological features, and neurological outcome, were assessed and further analyzed. Outcome was assessed according to the modified Rankin scale (mRS) at 6 months and stratified into favorable (mRS 0–2) versus unfavorable (mRS 3–6). For retrospective analysis of our changed therapeutic regime, patients not meeting the inclusion criteria of the IMCVS trial were excluded for further analysis.

2.3. Inclusion Criteria

Patient aged 18–75 years. Patients with aneurysmal SAH WFNS grades I-IV with hemodynamically relevant CVS defined as: 1. elevated time to peak (TTP) > 2 s compared to the corresponding contralateral side, or mean transit time (MTT) > 3.5 s; 2. profound narrowing of cerebral vessels of at least 50% in CT-A scan, especially in bilateral CVS; and 3. existence of "tissue at risk" (vital brain tissue with ischemic lesions <50%).

2.4. Induced Hypertension

Arterial hypertension, with a targeted mean arterial blood pressure (MAP) of 110 mmHg, was induced with norepinephrine and fluids via the central venous line. Induced hypertension was continued for 7 days. Thereafter, patients were re-assessed for CVS using CT-A/CT-P. In patients with persistent CVS, induced hypertension was continued for the following 7 days, and re-assessment was performed thereafter as described above. In patients with resolution of CVS, induced hypertension was terminated.

Invasive endovascular treatment (i.e., selective intraarterial infusion of vasodilators, or balloon angioplasty) was not performed at any timepoint (neither planned at a defined timepoint, nor as a rescue therapy).

2.5. Primary and Secondary Endpoints

The imaging data for new infarctions during the phase of CVS were assessed. The flow chart of the diagnostic protocol and the efficacy assessment are published in Vatter et al., 2011 [3].

The imaging data for new infarctions during the phase of CVS were assessed by a neuroradiologist blinded for treatment allocation. The cerebrum was partitioned into 19 segments. A 50% ischemic lesion $\geq$ 1 segment was defined as major, and <50% was defined as a minor infarct.

The primary outcome measure was the development of new cerebral infarctions during the phase of CVS. Secondary endpoints included clinical outcome at 6 months after SAH according to the modified Rankin scale (mRs).

2.6. Statistics

Data analysis was performed using the computer software package R (4.1.0). Comparisons between two groups in ordinal or continuous variables were conducted by Monte Carlo Mann–Whitney U tests. Two groups within nominal variables were compared by Monte Carlo chi-square tests. The number of repetitions in all Monte Carlo tests was set to 10^6. The Monte Carlo variants [4] of the statistical tests were necessary because ordinal variables had many ties and contingency tables had sometimes too few cell frequencies. In those cases, the asymptotic distribution was not reliable. In multivariate analysis, the first logistic regression was used to estimate the covariate between DCI and the covariates CVS, clinical vasospasm, smoking, WFNS grade, sex, age, and re-bleeding before treatment. The second logistic regression modeled the response indicator of mRS score >3 by the covariate's indicator of WFNS grades $\geq$ 3, minor and major DCI, re-bleeding before and after treatment, age, clinical vasospasm, and smoking. Before fitting the final multivariate regression models, a backward variable selection based on the AIC criterion was used.

3. Results

3.1. Patient Characteristics

We analyzed 303 patients with SAH (WFNS grades I-IV) treated in the authors' institution; 149 patients (49.2%) developed CVS and were treated with induced hypertension.

Of the 149 patients with CVS, 35 patients experienced DCI (23.5%, Table 1). Of these, 11 patients had a concomitant delayed ischemic neurologic deficit (31.4%, DIND), and 24 patients had no evidence of DIND.

Table 1. Patient characteristics.

Variable	DCI (n = 35)	No DCI (n = 114)	p-Value
Age, Y ± SD, mean	54 ± 11	55 ± 14	0.2
Female gender (%)	22 (63)	66 (58)	0.6
Smoker (%)	14 (40)	52 (46)	0.9
mRS before SAH	0	0	0.9
Hydrocephalus at admission (%)	27 (77.1)	73 (64)	1.0
WFNS grade	2 ± 1	2 ± 1	0.9
Fisher score	3	3	0.9
IVH	8	34	1.0
ICH < 3 cm	2	15	0.1
ICH > 3 cm	0	4	0.1
Aneurysm size	6 ± 3	7 ± 4	0.051
Warning leak	1	5	0.4
Coiling/Clipping	23/12	49/65	0.02
mRs ≤ 3 after 6 months	13 (37.1%)	81 (71%)	<0.001

ICH = intracerebral hemorrhage; IVH = intraventricular hemorrhage; mRS = modified Rankin scale; SAH = subarachnoid hemorrhage; Y = years.

3.2. Aneurysm Treatment

In total, 153 patients were treated by coiling, and 150 patients by clipping.

3.3. Rebleeding

Six of the 303 SAH (1.9%) patients experienced early re-bleeding after aneurysm treatment. Five of the six patients with re-bleeding after treatment had been treated with coiling, and one with clipping.

3.4. Delayed Cerebral Ischemia

A CVS-related minor infarction was found in 18 patients, and a major infarction in 17 patients.

Nine of the 11 patients (81.8%) with CVS and concomitant DIND developed DCI. Five of the 11 patients (45.4%) with concomitant DIND developed a minor infarction, and 4 of the 11 patients (36.4%) developed a major infarction.

3.5. Outcome

In total, 81 of the 114 patients (71%) without DCI, compared to 13 of 35 patients (37.1%) with DCI, achieved favorable outcomes (mRs ≤ 3) after 6 months.

3.6. Multivariate Analyses

Of those variables analyzed for influence on the development of DCI in the univariate analyses, the variable "CVS" ($p = 0.001$; odds ratio (OR) = 26; 95% confidence interval (CI) 3.3–209) remained significant in the multivariate model (Nagelkerke's $R^2 = 0.32$). In the multivariate regression model, the variables "DIND", "smoker", "WFNS-grades", "endovasular treatment", "gender", and "re-bleeding before treatment" were eliminated from the model.

In a second multivariate model, we analyzed variables that are known to influence clinical outcome. Of the variables that influenced poor outcome (mRs >3), the variables "WFNS grade 3–4" ($p = 0.001$; OR = 6.2; 95% CI 2.6–15), "re-bleeding before treatment" ($p = 0.001$; OR = 24.2; 95% CI 3.5–165), "DCI- minor infarction" ($p = 0.006$; OR = 4.7; 95% CI 1.6–14.6), and "DCI- major infarction" ($p = 0.001$; OR = 12.2; 95% CI 3.6–41) remained significant in the multivariate model (Nagelkerke's $R^2 = 0.43$). In the multivariate regression model, the variables "age", "DIND", "endovascular treatment", "smoker", and "re-bleeding after treatment" were eliminated from the model (Table 2).

Table 2. Multivariate analyses.

Variable	OR	CI	p-Value
Multivariate analysis: Predictors of DCI (Nagelkerke's R^2 = 0.32)			
CVS	26	3.3–209	**0.001**
DIND	2.5	0.06–5.3	0.6
Smoker	4	0.3–64	0.3
WFNS-grades	2.4	0.4–18	0.4
Endovascular treatment	1.3	0.6–2.6	0.4
Gender	2.5	0.4–15	0.3
Re-bleeding before treatment	2.5	0.06–104	0.6
Multivariate analysis: Predictors of poor outcome (Nagelkerke's R^2 = 0.43)			
WFNS grade 3–4	6.2	2.6–15	**0.001**
Re-bleeding before treatment	24.2	3.5–165	**0.001**
DCI-minor infarction	4.7	1.6–14.6	**0.006**
DCI-major infarction	12.2	3.6–41	**0.001**
Age	0.96	0.93–1.1	0.09
DIND	2	0.9–4.6	0.1
Endovascular treatment	0.5	0.08–3.7	0.5
Smoker	1.2	0.5–3	0.7
Re-bleeding after treatment	4.8	0.6–38	0.1

CI = 95% confidence interval; CVS = cerebral vasospasm; DCI = delayed cerebral ischemia; DIND = delayed ischemic neurologic deficit; OR = odds ratio; WFNS = World Federation of Neurosurgical Societies; p-values < 0.05 are marked bold.

4. Discussion

In the present study of SAH patients with clearly defined assessment of CVS and its therapeutic management with induced hypertension, 23.5% of SAH patients with CVS being at high risk for DCI experienced DCI, while 76.5% did not.

Despite its widespread use, there is currently no evidence that invasive endovascular therapy decreases DCI rates or improves outcome in patients with SAH. Procedure-related complications seem to outrank its benefits [5]. After the prospective IMCVS trial that failed to demonstrate a benefit from invasive endovascular rescue therapy in SAH patients with CVS, we changed our treatment policy to induced hypertension only in patients with SAH and diagnosed CVS. DCI rates vary in this vulnerable patient population suffering from CVS.

The prospective randomized trial, hypertension induction in the management of aneurysmal subarachnoid hemorrhage with secondary ischaemia (HIMALAIA) [6], did not support induced hypertension for the management of CVS. However, it was underpowered to draw definitive conclusions. Haegens et al. [7] analyzed SAH patients with diagnosed CVS retrospectively and compared DCI rates in the group of patients with induced hypertension and without. They found DCI rates of 20% in the induced hypertension group compared to 33% in the group without induced hypertension, concluding that induced hypertension seems to be effective in the prevention of DCI and consecutive poor outcome. These DCI rates of 20% in the induced hypertension group are comparable to the DCI rates of the present study (23.5%).

Jabbarli et al. [8] compared two cohorts of SAH patients with CVS/DIND treated either early or delayed with endovascular therapy and found that patients in the early treatment group experienced DCI in 20.8% versus in 29% in the group of delayed endovascular treatment. The rate of DCI in the early endovascular intervention group was similar to the DCI rates of the induced hypertension group of the present study. However, while the DCI rates are not different, any form of additional therapy may increase the rate of unintended complications. Unfortunately, complication rates are not given in all published studies. Adami et al. [5] evaluated complication rates of selective intraarterial infusion of nimodipine and percutaneous transluminal balloon angioplasty (TBA). They found new infarctions in 53% of the patients', including 11% of patients with new infarctions that were deemed procedure-related, directly attributable to endovascular treatment (e.g., embolic complications and iatrogenic dissection). Labeyrie et al. [9] published a series of 145 patients who underwent angioplasty for CVS. They found intracranial dissections in 8%, intracranial embolism in 5%, worsening of CVS in 8%, and reperfusion syndrome with and without intracerebral hemorrhage in 5%. The study also failed to prove a clinical benefit of angioplasty in the SAH population. Additionally, to directly attributable complications, any kind of intrahospital transport for diagnostics and intervention bears the risk of transport-related complications, e.g., drop in blood pressure and lowering of blood supply below demand, resulting in ischemia. Furthermore, Hosmann et al. [10] found detrimental effects of intrahospital transports on cerebral metabolism in patients with SAH, leading to sustained impaired neuronal metabolism for several hours. The authors concluded that any kind of intrahospital transport for neuro-imaging should strongly be reconsidered and only indicated if the expected benefits outweigh the risks. It is intuitive that this also holds true for the vulnerable patient population with SAH and additional CVS.

Induced hypertension in patients with SAH and proven CVS decreases DCI rates to 20–24% (Haegens et al., and present study) [7]. The intervention is performed bedside without the necessity of repetitive intrahospital transports. Failure to respond to induced hypertension in patients with symptomatic vasospasm leads to a higher rate of cerebral infarction and poor outcome after 1 year compared to the group of patients who respond to induced hypertension [11].

In conclusion, possible benefits of any additional therapy for SAH patients with CVS treated with induced hypertension may be limited to a certain subgroup. Unfortunately, it is unclear which patient cohort this subgroup would be.

In the present study, the rate of DCI was higher in the group of patients treated endovascularly, compared to the group of patients treated surgically. While this result is surprising, it may only reflect a different distribution of known risk factors for the development of DCI, e.g., amount of cisternal and intraventricular blood, between the treatment groups. Due to the fact that treatment allocation was neither stratified according to the risk factors for DCI between the treatment groups nor randomized, no further conclusions can be drawn concerning the effect of treatment modality on DCI.

Limitations

The most obvious limitation is the retrospective design of the study. However, after the failed IMCVS trial led by the senior author of the present study, the intention was to prospectively follow the changed treatment policy of induced hypertension only and its results. Further benefits of the study are the clear definition and screening of CVS using CT-A/CT-P at days 6–8 after SAH. By analyzing rates of DCI, however, it is clear that by including high- and low-grade SAH patients the assessments of neurological status in awake and sedated patients may have been different.

5. Conclusions

In conclusion, we found that the omittance of invasive endovascular rescue therapies, additional to induced hypertension, in SAH patients with CVS does not lead to a higher rate of delayed cerebral ischemia compared to data from the literature and to data of the conservative treatment group of the IMCVS trial. Potential benefits of additional endovascular treatment for CVS need to be addressed in further studies, searching for a subgroup of patients who may benefit.

Author Contributions: Conceptualization E.G. and H.V.; methodology E.G., H.V. and T.W.; data curation E.G., T.L., A.G. and S.B.; writing—original draft preparation E.G. and H.V. writing—review and editing, H.V., J.W., F.D., F.L., A.G., M.V. and E.G.; visualization E.G. and J.W.; supervision E.G. and H.V. All authors have read and agreed to the published version of the manuscript.

Funding: This research received no external funding.

Institutional Review Board Statement: The study was conducted according to the guidelines of the Declaration of Helsinki and approved by the Ethics Committee of the Medical Faculty and the University Hospital of Bonn (code: 331/12).

Informed Consent Statement: Written informed consent was not needed because of the retrospective design. Local ethics committee waived patient informed consent for this retrospective observational study.

Data Availability Statement: All data are included in this manuscript.

Conflicts of Interest: The authors declare no conflict of interest.

References

1. Roos, Y.B.; de Haan, R.J.; Beenen, L.F.; Groen, R.J.; Albrecht, K.W.; Vermeulen, M. Complications and outcome in patients with aneurysmal subarachnoid haemorrhage: A prospective hospital based cohort study in the Netherlands. *J. Neurol. Neurosurg. Psychiatry* **2000**, *68*, 337–341. [CrossRef] [PubMed]
2. Connolly, E.S., Jr.; Rabinstein, A.A.; Carhuapoma, J.R.; Derdeyn, C.P.; Dion, J.; Higashida, R.T.; Hoh, B.L.; Kirkness, C.J.; Naidech, A.M.; Ogilvy, C.S.; et al. Guidelines for the management of aneurysmal subarachnoid hemorrhage: A guideline for healthcare professionals from the American Heart Association/american Stroke Association. *Stroke* **2012**, *43*, 1711–1737. [CrossRef] [PubMed]
3. Vatter, H.; Güresir, E.; Berkefeld, J.; Beck, J.; Raabe, A.; Rochemont, R.D.M.D.; Seifert, V.; Weidauer, S. Perfusion-diffusion mismatch in MRI to indicate endovascular treatment of cerebral vasospasm after subarachnoid haemorrhage. *J. Neurol. Neurosurg. Psychiatry* **2011**, *82*, 876–883. [CrossRef] [PubMed]
4. Zhu, L.X. *Nonparametric Monte Carlo Tests and Their Applications*, 1st ed.; Springer: Berlin/Heidelberg, Germany, 2005.
5. Adami, D.; Berkefeld, J.; Platz, J.; Konczalla, J.; Pfeilschifter, W.; Weidauer, S.; Wagner, M. Complication rate of intraarterial treatment of severe cerebral vasospasm after subarachnoid hemorrhage with nimodipine and percutaneous transluminal balloon angioplasty: Worth the risk? *J. Neuroradiol.* **2019**, *46*, 15–24. [CrossRef] [PubMed]
6. Gathier, C.S.; van den Bergh, W.M.; van der Jagt, M.; Verweij, B.H.; Dankbaar, J.W.; Müller, M.C.; Oldenbeuving, A.W.; Rinkel, G.J.E.; Slooter, A.J.C.; HIMALAIA Study Group. Induced Hypertension for Delayed Cerebral Ischemia After Aneurysmal Subarachnoid Hemorrhage: A Randomized Clinical Trial. *Stroke* **2018**, *49*, 76–83. [CrossRef] [PubMed]
7. Haegens, N.M.; Gathier, C.S.; Horn, J.; Coert, B.A.; Verbaan, D.; van den Bergh, W.M. Induced Hypertension in Preventing Cerebral Infarction in Delayed Cerebral Ischemia After Subarachnoid Hemorrhage. *Stroke* **2018**, *49*, 2630–2636. [CrossRef] [PubMed]
8. Jabbarli, R.; Pierscianek, D.; Rölz, R.; Oppong, M.D.; Kaier, K.; Shah, M.; Taschner, C.; Mönninghoff, C.; Urbach, H.; Beck, J.; et al. Endovascular treatment of cerebral vasospasm after subarachnoid hemorrhage: More is more. *Neurology* **2019**, *93*, e458–e466. [CrossRef] [PubMed]
9. Labeyrie, M.-A.; Gaugain, S.; Boulouis, G.; Zetchi, A.; Brami, J.; Saint-Maurice, J.-P.; Civelli, V.; Froelich, S.; Houdart, E. Distal Balloon Angioplasty of Cerebral Vasospasm Decreases the Risk of Delayed Cerebral Infarction. *AJNR Am. J. Neuoradiol.* **2019**, *40*, 1342–1348. [CrossRef] [PubMed]
10. Hosmann, A.; Angelmayr, C.; Hopf, A.; Rauscher, S.; Brugger, J.; Ritscher, L.; Bohl, I.; Schnackenburg, P.; Engel, A.; Plöchl, W.; et al. Detrimental effects of intrahospital transport on cerebral metabolism in patients suffering severe aneurysmal subarachnoid hemorrhage. *J. Neurosurg.* **2021**, 1–8. [CrossRef] [PubMed]
11. Suwatcharangkoon, S.; De Marchis, G.M.; Witsch, J.; Meyers, E.; Velazquez, A.; Falo, C.; Schmidt, J.M.; Agarwal, S.; Connolly, E.S.; Claassen, J.; et al. Medical Treatment Failure for Symptomatic Vasospasm After Subarachnoid Hemorrhage Threatens Long-Term Outcome. *Stroke* **2019**, *50*, 1696–1702. [CrossRef] [PubMed]

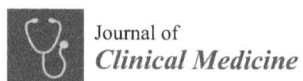

Article

Impact of Anemia Severity on the Outcome of an Aneurysmal Subarachnoid Hemorrhage

Maryam Said [1,2,*], Thiemo Florin Dinger [1,2], Meltem Gümüs [1,2], Laurèl Rauschenbach [1,2], Mehdi Chihi [1,2], Jan Rodemerk [1,2], Veronika Lenz [3], Marvin Darkwah Oppong [1,2], Anne-Kathrin Uerschels [1,2], Philipp Dammann [1,2], Karsten Henning Wrede [1,2], Ulrich Sure [1,2] and Ramazan Jabbarli [1,2]

1 Department of Neurosurgery and Spine Surgery, University Hospital of Essen, 45147 Essen, Germany
2 Center for Translational Neuro- and Behavioral Sciences (C-TNBS), University Duisburg Essen, 47147 Duisburg, Germany
3 Institute of Transfusion Medicine, University Hospital of Essen, 45147 Essen, Germany
* Correspondence: maryam.said@uk-essen.de; Tel.: +49-201-723-1201; Fax: +49-201-723-5909

Abstract: Objective: Previous reports indicate a negative impact of anemia on the outcome of an aneurysmal subarachnoid hemorrhage (SAH). We aimed to identify the outcome-relevant severity of post-SAH anemia. Methods: SAH cases treated at our institution between 01/2005 and 06/2016 were included ($n = 640$). The onset, duration, and severity (nadir hemoglobin (nHB) level) of anemia during the initial hospital stay were recorded. Study endpoints were new cerebral infarctions, a poor outcome six months post-SAH (modified Rankin scale > 3), and in-hospital mortality. To assess independent associations with the study endpoints, different multivariable regression models were performed, adjusted for relevant patient and baseline SAH characteristics as well as anemia-associated clinical events during the SAH. Results: The rates of anemia were 83.3%, 67.7%, 40.0%, 15.9%, and 4.5% for an nHB < 11 g/dL, < 10 g/dL, < 9 g/dL, < 8 g/dL, and < 7 g/dL, respectively. The higher the anemia severity, the later was the onset (post-SAH days 2, 4, 5.4, 7.6 and 8, $p < 0.0001$) and the shorter the duration (8 days, 6 days, 4 days, 3 days, and 2 days, $p < 0.0001$) of anemia. In the final multivariable analysis, only an nHB < 9 g/dL was independently associated with all study endpoints: adjusted odds ratio 1.7/3.22/2.44 for cerebral infarctions/in-hospital mortality/poor outcome. The timing (post-SAH day 3.9 vs. 6, $p = 0.001$) and duration (3 vs. 5 days, $p = 0.041$) of anemia with an nHB < 9 g/dL showed inverse associations with the risk of in-hospital mortality, but not with other study endpoints. Conclusions: Anemia is very common in SAH patients affecting four of five individuals during their hospital stay. An nHB decline to < 9 g/dL was strongly associated with all study endpoints, independent of baseline characteristics and SAH-related clinical events. Our data encourage further prospective evaluations of the value of different transfusion strategies in the functional outcomes of SAH patients.

Keywords: subarachnoid hemorrhage; anemia; outcome; risk factors

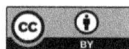

1. Introduction

Anemia is a common condition after an acute aneurysmal subarachnoid hemorrhage (SAH). Although often based on small case series, existing reports indicate a negative impact of anemia on the outcome in SAH patients [1–3].

A decline in hemoglobin (Hb) value during a SAH has repeatedly been described, often in the context of aneurysm surgery and conservative management of delayed cerebral ischemia [4]. Associations between Hb decline and poorer clinical condition, longer hospital stay, unfavorable outcome, and increased mortality have been reported [5,6]. Despite these findings, there are no specific guidelines or recommendations for managing anemia during a SAH. In fact, in the current literature, the cut-off Hb value for anemia, and with that the threshold for its treatment, varies greatly [7,8]. In addition, it remains unclear whether anemia has an independent impact on SAH outcome or is the consequence of poor initial clinical condition or specific complications during a SAH, such as aneurysm rebleeding, cerebral vasospasm, or systemic infections. Finally, insufficient and inconsistent data are available on the significance of the onset and duration of anemia in the context of its clinical impact.

In our large monocentric observational cohort study, we aimed to analyze the occurrence, time trends, and clinical impact of post-SAH anemia, with a particular emphasis on identifying outcome-relevant anemia severity.

2. Materials and Methods

2.1. Patient Population

For this retrospective study, all patients aged 18 years and older treated for an aneurysmal SAH at our institution between January 2005 and June 2016 were considered eligible. Exclusion criteria for this study were: (1) no treatment for the SAH was received, (2) late admission (> 48 h after ictus), and (3) pre-existing anemia in the context of another disease. The study was registered in the German trial registry (DRKS, Unique identifier: RKS00008749) and approved by the local ethics committee (Ethik-Kommission, Medizinische Fakultät der Universität Duisburg-Essen, Registration number: 15-6331-BO).

2.2. SAH Management

The bleeding source was diagnosed using digital subtraction angiography (DSA) in all patients who presented at our institution with a suspected SAH. After a ruptured intracranial aneurysm was confirmed, microsurgical clipping or endovascular coiling and/or stenting was commonly performed within 24 h after admission.

Conservative management included oral nimodipine for 21 days and the maintenance of normovolemia and mean arterial pressure > 70 mmHg. Vasospasm surveillance consisted of daily neurological assessment and transcranial Doppler ultrasound (TCD). In addition, patients underwent repeated DSAs for the identification and, if confirmed, endovascular treatment of vasospasm [9] in the following cases: (1) neurological worsening, defined as a new neurological deficit or a ≥ 2 points decline in the Glasgow coma scale not attributable to other complications (such as rebleeding or hydrocephalus); (2) in unconscious patients, development of absolute mean flow velocities > 120 cm/s or an increase of more than 50% compared to the previous measurement in TCD. In the SAH patients with clinical and/or angiographic signs of cerebral vasospasm, conservative management was escalated by increasing the target mean arterial pressure to > 90 mmHg.

Acute hydrocephalus was treated with an external ventricular drain. This device also allowed for continuous intracranial pressure (ICP) monitoring. In cases of pathologically increased ICP (> 20 mmHg) refractory to conservative management [10], decompressive craniectomy (DC) was performed.

Regular laboratory measurements, performed three times weekly for at least 14 days after ictus, assessed anemia occurrence during the SAH, with an increased frequency of blood sampling if clinically indicated. According to the institutional standards based on the widely accepted recommendation for critical care patients [11], red blood cell transfusion (RBCT) was performed in case of a decrease in nadir Hb (nHb) to < 7.0 g/dL.

Computed tomography (CT) scans were performed at admission, within 24 h after aneurysm treatment (or any other neurosurgical procedure), in case of neurological deterioration, and during weaning from external ventricular drainage. There were no significant changes in the institutional SAH management protocol during the reported years.

2.3. Data Management

Anemia severity was assessed according to the nHb levels which were documented during the 14 days after the SAH at predefined cutoffs: < 11 g/dL, < 10 g/dL, < 9 g/dL, < 8 g/dL, and < 7 g/dL. The onset (since ictus, in days) and duration (number of days with each nHb level) of anemia were also documented. Furthermore, data on patients' demographic characteristics, previous comorbidities and regular medication, initial SAH severity, and treatment modality, and on the occurrence of certain adverse events, were collected from the institutional retrospective aneurysm database. The patients' initial clinical condition was recorded using the World Federation of Neurosurgical Societies (WFNS) scale [12], with further dichotomization into good (WFNS = 1–3) and poor (WFNS = 4–5) grades. Furthermore, radiographic severity was graded according to the original Fisher scale [13], which was also dichotomized (grade 3–4 vs. 1–2) for further analysis. The following complications during the SAH were recorded: aneurysm rebleeding, cerebral vasospasm (based on the presence of the above-mentioned neurologic and/or angiographic characteristics), ICP increase necessitating DC, acute coronary syndrome (ACS), and systemic infections. Finally, functional outcome was assessed at discharge and 6 months after the SAH using the modified Rankin scale (mRS) [14], with an mRS > 3 regarded as an unfavorable outcome.

2.4. Study Endpoints and Statistical Analyses

As the primary study endpoints, we investigated the impact of post-SAH anemia severity on the occurrence of the following major outcome events: (1) occurrence of cerebral infarction(s); (2) in-hospital mortality; (3) unfavorable outcome at 6 months post-SAH. The associations between each nHb level and all three outcome events were tested using a univariate analysis and two models of a multivariable binary logistic regression analysis. The univariate analysis was based on the chi-squared or Fisher's exact test, as appropriate. In the multivariable analysis, the first model (M1) included the following confounders: patients' age (dichotomized at the cohort's mean age), sex, WFNS and Fisher grades at admission, presence of acute hydrocephalus, and length of hospital stay. Along with all covariates from the M1 model, the second model (M2) of the multivariable analysis was enhanced by adverse events during the SAH which were significantly associated with the occurrence of anemia and the primary outcome endpoints.

Furthermore, the following analyses were also performed as the secondary study endpoints: (a) the relationship between anemia severity with its onset and duration; (b) the impact of the onset and/or duration of the outcome-relevant anemia severity on the above-mentioned major outcome events; (c) the associations between patients' baseline and SAH characteristics with the severity of post-SAH anemia. For normally distributed continuous variables, analyses were performed with the Student's t-test. Non-normally distributed continuous variables were analyzed with the Mann-Whitney U-test and one-way ANOVA, as required. The missing values were replaced by multiple imputations. Data analysis was performed using SPSS statistical software (version 27.0). Correlations with a p-value of < 0.05 were considered statistically significant.

2.5. Data Availability Statement

Any data not published within the article will be shared in an anonymized manner on request with any qualified investigator.

3. Results

After excluding non-eligible cases (no aneurysm treatment: n = 33; late admission: n = 96; pre-existing anemia: n = 9), a total of 640 patients were included in the final analyses. The baseline characteristics of the cohort are presented in Table 1.

Table 1. Baseline characteristics of the final cohort.

Parameter	Number of Cases	Percentage *
Demographic characteristics and previous medical history		
Age ≥ 55	297	46.4%
Female sex	420	65.6%
Ethnicity (non-Caucasian)	28	4.4%

Table 1. Cont.

Parameter	Number of Cases	Percentage *
Hypertension	454	71.0%
Hypothyroidism	81	12.7%
Hyperthyroidism	5	0.8%
Hypercholesterolemia	53	8.4%
Hyperuricemia	18	2.9%
Diabetes mellitus Type II	38	6.0%
Statins	35	5.6%
Chronic painkiller abuse	47	7.5%
Blood thinners	56	8.8%
Initial characteristics of the SAH		
WFNS Grade (4–5)	283	44.2%
Fisher Grade (3–4)	532	88.8%
Acute hydrocephalus	488	76.3%
Aneurysm rebleed	31	4.8%
Clipping	262	40.9%
Aneurysm location ICA MCA AcoA ACA PC	67 152 230 22 169	10.4% 23.8% 35.9% 3.4% 26.4%
Aneurysm sack ≥ 7 mm	294	46.8%
Adverse events during the SAH		
Decompressive craniectomy	196	30.6%
Sonographic vasospasms	306	52.7%
Angiographically treated vasospasms	178	27.8%
Acute coronary syndrome	17	3.0%
Systemic infections	264	45.0%

Abbreviations: WFNS = World Federation of Neurosurgical Societies, ICA = internal carotid artery, MCA = middle cerebral artery, AcoA = anterior communicating artery, ACA = anterior cerebral artery, PC = posterior circulation. *—the percentages for each parameter were calculated according to the number of cases with known values.

3.1. Post-SAH Anemia: The Prevalence and Timing

There was a decreasing rate of anemia in the cohort, depending on its severity. The lower the documented nHb value during the first two weeks of SAH treatment, the less frequent was the rate of anemia severity (Figure 1). In particular, a decrease of nHb to < 11.0 g/dL was very common in our SAH cohort, affecting a little more than four out of five SAH patients. On the other hand, the most severe anemia with an nHb < 7.0 g/dL was a sporadic condition observed in < 5% of the cohort.

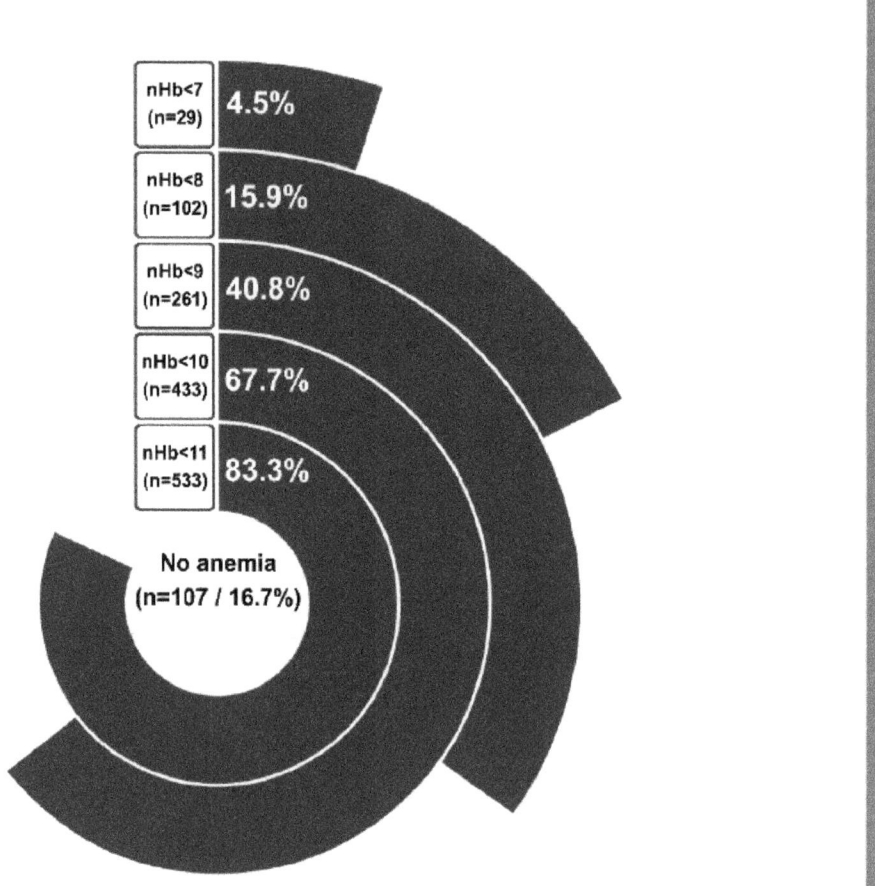

Figure 1. All patients in the cohort are represented based on the nadir Hb (nHb) level. For every anemia subgroup the number of patients and percentage of the total population are depicted, respectively.

There was also a significant association between the onset of the anemia and its severity (Figure 2). With increasing anemia severity, a later onset in the course of the SAH was observed: on post-SAH days 2, 4, 5.4, 7.6, and 8 for an nHb < 11.0 g/dL, < 10.0 g/dL, < 9.0 g/dL, < 8.0 g/dL, and < 7.0 g/dL, respectively ($p < 0.0001$). Of notice, the number of days patients suffered from anemia was also significantly dependent on its severity. On average, an nHb < 7.0 g/dL lasted for no more than 2 days, whereas an nHb < 11.0 g/dL was seen for considerably longer in patients (mean: 8 days, 6 days, 4 days, 3 days, and 2 days for an nHb < 11.0 g/dL, < 10.0 g/dL, < 9.0 g/dL, < 8.0 g/dL, and < 7.0 g/dL, respectively, $p < 0.0001$).

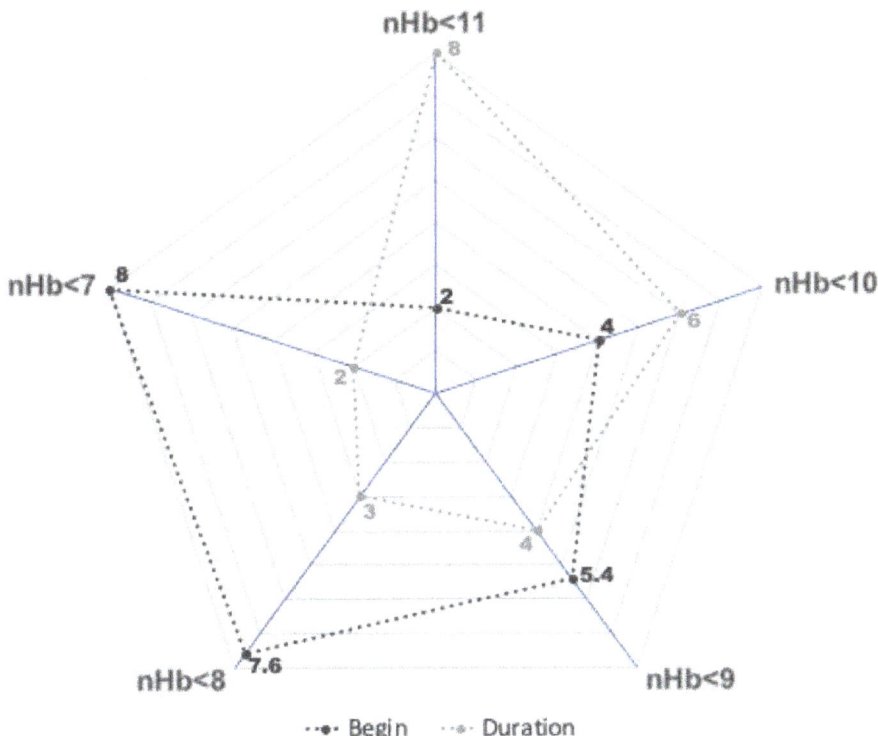

Figure 2. Onset and duration of anemia in days for each subgroup of anemia. For every g/dL drop in nadir hemoglobin (nHb) level, a later onset during the SAH was observed. The duration of the anemia was inversely related to its severity.

3.2. Prognostic Factors for Post-SAH Anemia

Table 2 presents the summary of the odds ratios for the associations between patients' baseline and initial SAH characteristics along with the occurrence of post-SAH anemia at different nHb cut-offs (see Supplementary Table S1 for more detailed data on the performed univariate analysis). Patients aged 55 years and older had a significantly higher risk of developing anemia (nHb < 8.0 g/dL, < 9.0 g/dL, and < 10.0 g/dL) during the SAH. Female sex was also significantly correlated with an nHb < 10.0 g/dL and < 11.0 g/dL. Regarding previous medical history, arterial hypertension (nHb < 8 g/dL and < 9.0 g/dL), hypercholesterinemia (nHb < 10.0 g/dL), diabetes mellitus (nHb < 10.0 g/dL and < 11.0 g/dL), and treatment with statins (nHb < 10.0 g/dL) increased the probability of anemia at different severity levels. Furthermore, the initial severity of the SAH (high WFNS and Fisher scales and the presence of acute hydrocephalus) showed robust associations with the risk of anemia during the SAH, with significance observed for a wide range of documented nHb values (between < 8.0 g/dL and 11.0 g/dL). Finally, the following clinical events during the SAH were also linked with the occurrence of anemia at different severity levels: surgical treatment with clipping and/or DC (for an nHb < 8.0 g/dL, < 9.0 g/dL, < 10.0 g/dL, and < 11.0 g/dL), cerebral vasospasm (nHb < 9.0 g/dL, < 10.0 g/dL, and < 11.0 g/dL), ACS (nHb < 8.0 g/dL), and systemic infections (nHb between < 8.0 g/dL and < 11.0 g/dL). Interestingly, aneurysm rebleeding before treatment did not impact the probability of post-SAH anemia.

Table 2. Univariate analyses of baseline characteristics as predictors of anemia in SAH.

Hb Variable / Nadir	< 7.0 g/dL	< 8.0 g/dL	< 9.0 g/dL	< 10.0 g/dL	< 11.0 g/dL
	OR (95% CI)				
Demographic parameters and comorbidities					
Age ≥ 55 years	1.95 (0.90–4.19)	**1.81 (1.18–2.79)**	**1.87 (1.36–2.57)**	**1.42 (1.01–1.98)**	1.36 (0.89–2.07)
Female sex	0.85 (0.40–1.84)	0.86 (0.56–1.34)	1.11 (0.80–1.55)	**1.54 (1.09–2.17)**	**2.36 (1.55–3.60)**
Ethnicity (non-Caucasian)	0.77 (0.10–5.89)	1.47 (0.58–3.71)	1.27 (0.60–2.72)	1.79 (0.72–4.49)	1.71 (0.51–5.76)
Hypertension	1.59 (0.64–3.98)	**1.82 (1.08–3.07)**	**1.45 (1.02–2.07)**	1.33 (0.93–1.91)	1.07 (0.68–1.69)
Hypercholesterolemia	1.27 (0.37–4.36)	1.59 (0.80–3.14)	1.34 (0.76–2.36)	**2.51 (1.20–5.24)**	2.03 (0.79–5.23)
Hypothyroidism	1.59 (0.59–4.29)	1.10 (0.58–2.09)	1.06 (0.66–1.73)	1.62 (0.93–2.83)	1.37 (0.68–2.76)
Hyperthyroidism	1.87 (0.10–34.63)	0.47 (0.03–8.63)	2.19 (0.36–13.21)	1.92 (0.21–17.29)	2.24 (0.12–40.79)
Hyperuricemia	2.71 (0.59–12.40)	2.05 (0.71–5.87)	1.87 (0.73–4.79)	1.26 (0.44–3.58)	1.64 (0.37–7.22)
Diabetes mellitus	1.18 (0.27–5.16)	1.20 (0.51–2.81)	1.49 (0.77–2.87)	**4.31 (1.51–12.33)**	**7.85 (1.07–57.84)**
Renal diseases	0.38 (0.02–6.47)	1.32 (0.48–3.58)	0.98 (0.43–2.21)	0.85 (0.37–1.96)	0.80 (0.29–2.18)
Regular medication					
Statins	1.38 (0.31–6.05)	1.68 (0.74–3.80)	1.24 (0.63–2.47)	**2.99 (1.14–7.83)**	2.17 (0.65–7.22)
Painkiller abuse	0.43 (0.06–3.24)	0.60 (0.23–1.57)	1.0 (0.55–1.83)	0.63 (0.34–1.15)	0.73 (0.35–1.52)
Blood thinners	2.28 (0.84–6.24)	1.49 (0.76–2.94)	1.39 (0.80–2.41)	1.84 (0.95–3.57)	1.75 (0.73–4.18)
Initial SAH severity					
WFNS grade (4–5)	2.14 (0.99–4.60)	**2.85 (1.83–4.45)**	**3.03 (2.19–4.21)**	**3.18 (2.21–4.57)**	**3.27 (2.01–5.31)**
Fisher grade (3–4)	7.91 (0.48–131.0)	**4.76 (1.46–15.46)**	**2.58 (1.44–4.64)**	**1.87 (1.12–3.15)**	**2.14 (1.17–3.91)**
Acute hydrocephalus	2.0 (0.68–5.83)	**3.30 (1.67–6.51)**	**3.02 (1.98–4.60)**	**2.83 (1.94–4.12)**	**2.75 (1.77–4.26)**
Aneurysm size ≥ 7 mm	1.54 (0.72–3.32)	1.22 (0.80–1.87)	1.15 (0.83–1.58)	1.14 (0.81–1.59)	1.24 (0.81–1.89)
Clinical events and complications during the SAH					
Aneurysm rebleed	2.3 (0.66–8.04)	1.54 (0.65–3.66)	1.31 (0.64–2.67)	2.15 (0.87–5.30)	1.99 (0.59–6.65)
Vasospasm	1.63 (0.75–3.51)	1.44 (0.92–2.27)	**1.74 (1.23–2.47)**	**2.78 (1.82–4.26)**	**3.58 (1.91–6.71)**
DC	1.64 (0.77–3.50)	**2.71 (1.76–4.18)**	**3.09 (2.18–4.37)**	**5.32 (3.31–8.55)**	**7.85 (3.57–17.24)**
ACS	1.36 (0.17–10.7)	**3.0 (1.08–8.35)**	2.14 (0.80–5.71)	2.33 (0.66–8.20)	1.46 (0.33–6.49)
Systemic infection	0.91 (0.42–1.97)	**1.71 (1.11–2.63)**	**2.28 (1.63–3.18)**	**3.23 (2.20–4.75)**	**3.92 (2.27–6.77)**
Clipping	0.64 (0.29–1.42)	**1.79 (1.17–2.73)**	**2.44 (1.76–3.37)**	**4.22 (2.86–6.24)**	**6.99 (3.75–13.05)**

Abbreviations: Hb = hemoglobin, OR = odds ratio, CI = confidence interval, WFNS = World Federation of Neurosurgical Societies, DC = decompressive craniectomy, ACS = acute coronary syndrome. Significant results are in bold.

3.3. Severity of Anemia in Relation to Primary Study Endpoints

The more severe the post-SAH anemia was, the higher was the burden of cerebral infarctions, in-hospital mortality, and unfavorable outcome at six months after the SAH (Figure 3). Univariate analyses showed significant correlations for almost all anemia levels with the analyzed outcome events (see Table 3 with summary data on univariate and multivariate analyses; see Supplementary Table S2 with detailed analysis of the study endpoints). However, in the final multivariable analysis (M2 model), only an nHb < 9.0 g/dL (adjusted odds ratio (aOR): 1.70, 95% confidence interval (CI): 1.16–2.50, $p = 0.007$) and an nHb < 10.0 g/dL (aOR: 1.83, 95% CI:

1.19–2.81, p = 0.006) were independently associated with the risk of cerebral infarction. In both multivariable models (M1 and M2), shorter survival during hospitalization showed a strong link with post-SAH anemia for nHb levels between < 8.0 g/dL and < 11.0 g/dL. Finally, unfavorable outcome at six months was independently associated with an nHb < 8.0 g/dL (aOR: 2.21, 95% CI: 1.21–4.04, p = 0.01) and < 9.0 g/dL (aOR: 2.44, 95% CI: 1.57–3.79, p < 0.0001) in the enhanced multivariable analysis (M2 model). In summary, post-SAH anemia at < 9.0 g/dL was the only nHb value that showed robust and strong associations with all study endpoints, independently of patients' outcome- and anemia-relevant baseline parameters, initial SAH characteristics, and clinical events during treatment.

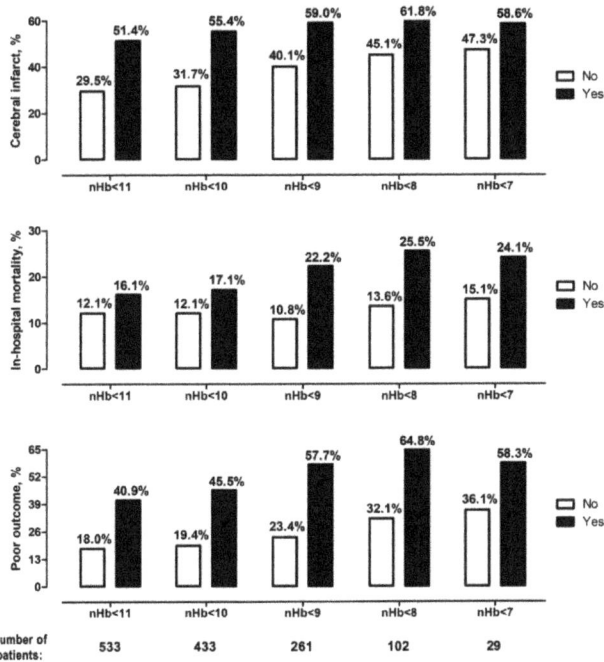

Figure 3. Occurrence of primary endpoints for the different degrees of anemia. There was a gradual increase in the rate of cerebral infarction, in-hospital mortality, and poor outcome for every nHb level decrease.

Table 3. Overview of univariate and multivariate analyses for every nadir Hb level.

Nadir Hb:		< 7.0 g/dL	< 8.0 g/dL	< 9.0 g/dL	< 10.0 g/dL	< 11.0 g/dL
Cerebral infarction	UVA	1.58 (0.74–3.36)	**1.96 (1.27–3.03)**	**2.15 (1.56–2.97)**	**2.68 (1.89–3.80)**	**2.53 (1.61–3.97)**
	MVA M1	1.29 (0.58–2.87)	1.54 (0.96–2.46)	**1.72 (1.21–2.46)**	**2.47 (1.66–3.68)**	**2.30 (1.38–3.84)**
	MVA M2	1.28 (0.56–2.96)	1.33 (0.82–2.17)	**1.70 (1.16–2.50)**	**1.83 (1.19–2.81)**	1.67 (0.98–2.86)
Unfavorable outcome at 6 months	UVA	**2.48 (1.08–5.68)**	**3.88 (2.41–6.25)**	**4.47 (3.13–6.39)**	**3.47 (2.31–5.23)**	**3.15 (1.84–5.42)**
	MVA M1	1.98 (0.80–4.92)	**2.85 (1.65–4.92)**	**3.05 (2.04–4.56)**	**2.19 (1.39–3.46)**	**2.17 (1.18–3.98)**
	MVA M2	1.98 (0.74–5.34)	**2.21 (1.21–4.04)**	**2.44 (1.57–3.79)**	1.50 (0.89–2.52)	1.43 (0.75–2.72)
In-hospital mortality	UVA	1.80 (0.75–4.32)	**2.18 (1.31–3.63)**	**2.36 (1.52–3.64)**	1.5 (0.92–2.44)	1.39 (0.75–2.60)
	MVA M1	2.43 (0.64–9.21)	**3.32 (1.62–7.23)**	**4.84 (2.49–9.41)**	**9.61 (4.08–22.62)**	**7.41 (2.74–20.04)**
	MVA M2	2.20 (0.50–9.68)	**2.44 (1.07–5.55)**	**3.22 (1.59–6.51)**	**6.06 (2.39–15.34)**	**4.60 (1.61–13.14)**

Abbreviations: UVA = univariate analysis, MVA = multivariate analysis, M1 = model 1, M2 = model 2. Significant findings (p < 0.05) are in bold.

When analyzing the value of the occurrence of an nHb < 9.0 g/dL for patients' outcome, the onset (post-SAH day 3.9 vs. 6, p = 0.001) and duration (3 days vs. 5 days, p = 0.041) of anemia showed inverse associations with the risk of in-hospital mortality, but not with the other study endpoints (see Supplementary Table S3).

4. Discussion

Anemia is a common finding in SAH patients. In our large observational study, we found that four out of five SAH patients suffered from anemia during their hospitalization. In previous literature, several degrees of anemia have been mentioned in relation to patients with SAH. Rates from 30% to almost 60% have been reported [15–18]. In our study, we found cerebral infarctions, in-hospital mortality, and poor neurological outcome to be independently associated with several degrees of anemia.

Although often described in this patient population, until now no common management strategies have been determined. The use of RBCT in this population is rather restrictive in most institutions [7,19–23]. A North American survey on RBCT practices found that the thresholds for transfusion vary between 7.0 g/dL and 10.0 g/dL [24]. Which RBCT threshold has the best risk–benefit profile for SAH patients is yet to be clarified, as RBCT has been associated with higher rates of thromboembolic events [23], poor outcome [25], vasospasm [26], and cognitive impairment [27].

To our knowledge, our study is the first to describe the occurrence, onset, and duration of a wide range of nHb levels within one large representative SAH cohort. The more severe the anemia, the later the onset in the course of disease. This association reflects the effect of the duration of neurocritical care treatment on the probability and severity of anemia. Therefore, duration of hospital stay is an essential parameter that should be considered in analyses evaluating the association between anemia and SAH outcome. In contrast to our study, where the length of hospitalization was incorporated in the statistical constructs, many previous studies failed to show robust associations between post-SAH anemia and in-hospital mortality [4,19,22,26,28].

Moreover, we were able to show that the more aggravating the anemia, the shorter its duration. This might be the consequence of both later anemia onset and the treating physicians' lower tolerance of more severe anemia grades. Only an nHb decrease to < 7.0 g/dL was an absolute indication for RBCT in our clinic. Accordingly, with an average of two days, nHb levels < 7.0 g/dL had the shortest duration in the cohort (compared to higher nHb values). Therefore, RBCT in SAH patients with nHb levels < 7.0 g/dL apparently resulted in swifter anemia correction than in SAH patients with less severe nHb levels. This circumstance might partially explain the less prominent link between an nHb < 7.0 g/dL and the study endpoints as compared to higher nHb levels which were tolerated longer than the standard institutional RBCT threshold of < 7.0 g/dL. Another possible explanation for the lack of significance of an nHb < 7.0 g/dL might be the small size of the subpopulation with this nHb, as only 4.5% of our cohort developed such a low nHb.

In our analysis, several baseline characteristics at admission were associated with the development of anemia in the course of the disease. Knowledge of these easily accessible parameters allows for early risk stratification and risk-adjusted anemia management, since many identified anemia predictors (such as patients' age and initial SAH severity) are also outcome-relevant prognostic factors for SAH patients [29]. Moreover, we found several premorbid conditions to be risk factors for developing post-SAH anemia. In particular, hypercholesterinemia (and statin treatment) and diabetes mellitus were associated with mild forms of anemia (< 10.0 g/dL and < 11.0 g/dL), and the presence of arterial hypertension was associated with an nHb decrease to < 8.0 g/dL and < 9.0 g/dL. There is no literature available on hypercholesterolemia and anemia in SAH patients, but a link between hypercholesterolemia and different chronic types of anemia has previously been described [30]. Patients with essential hypertension [31], and particularly those with pulmonary arterial hypertension [32], were reported to be at higher risk of anemia. Finally, diabetes-related chronic hyperglycemia can also lead to anemia via impaired erythropoietin production [33].

Even if the patient's previous medical history contributes to anemia risk to some extent, substantial post-SAH anemia is more likely triggered by several factors occurring during the course of the SAH disease. Along with common anemia confounders during intensive care treatment, such as phlebotomy and hemodilution [1,34], there are also SAH-specific clinical events which strongly increase the risk of acute anemia. In particular, surgical treatments, including aneurysm clipping and DC due to refractory ICP increase were significantly associated with anemia risk in our cohort. Both surgical factors had already been reported as anemia triggers in SAH patients [4,7,17]. Moreover, cerebral vasospasms and systemic infections also showed robust correlations with post-SAH anemia. The link between vasospasm and anemia was repeatedly reported in the context of SAH disease. However, the cause–effect relationship between these two events remains unclear; is the anemia the consequence of conservative vasospasm management [35], or should anemia rather be regarded as a marker of poor hemodynamic support, contributing to cerebral hypoxia and resulting in the clinical manifestation of cerebral vasospasm [36]? Or, alternatively, might these two SAH complications exist in a vicious circle? Finally, infections had also previously been reported as risk factors for the development of anemia in SAH patients [16,20]. In the context of intensive care unit treatment, systemic inflammation reduces red blood cell development by inhibiting erythropoietin synthesis, and it interferes with the ability of erythroblasts to incorporate iron [37,38].

A link between anemia and SAH outcome had already been shown in many previous studies [1,3,4,8,28,34,39]. However, these studies suffered from significant limitations with regard to different cut-off values for nHb and the uncertainty of whether anemia was independently related to SAH outcome or merely presented an epiphenomenon of the initial SAH severity and/or of clinical complications during SAH. In our analysis, we adjusted for patients' baseline characteristics, initial SAH severity, and outcome/anemia-relevant clinical events. We analyzed different nHb levels and found robust independent correlations between an nHb decrease to < 9.0 g/dL and the occurrence of cerebral infarctions, in-hospital mortality, and unfavorable outcome at six months. With the two MVA models we conducted for these analyses, we were able to correct for the hemodiluting effects of SAH therapy. This means that anemia is not in fact an epiphenomenon, but rather an independent predictor in SAH.

Our findings imply a higher RBCT threshold for SAH patients than is currently being practiced in our and many other neurovascular centers, where patients receive transfusions only in cases in which nHb decrease is < 7.0 g/dL. This restrictive transfusion policy is based on the largest to-date prospective clinical trial that evaluated the risks and benefits of RBCT in patients in the intensive care unit [11]. Of note, patients with a SAH were underrepresented in this study, published in 1999. This circumstance, along with the current data on the association between anemia and SAH outcome, necessitates the reconsideration of the current standards for RBCT in SAH patients. Therefore, we recommend a prospective evaluation of the value of different transfusion strategies in the functional outcomes of SAH patients.

5. Limitations

Our study has certain limitations, mainly its single-center and retrospective design. Moreover, there is an additional risk of selection and information bias, since the patients with a more aggravating course of illness tend to undergo more invasive procedures and have relatively more blood drawn for tests. Finally, our center does not use invasive monitoring of cerebral oxygenation. These data on the oxygen delivery in the effector tissue would be relevant for confirming the findings and hypotheses of this study. Nevertheless, the present study is based on a large representative SAH cohort. We utilized an extensive explorative analysis, addressing different nHb values with the adjustment of study results for the most relevant baseline patient and clinical characteristics and adverse events during the SAH.

6. Conclusions

We found anemia to be very common in SAH patients, affecting four in five individuals during their hospital stay. Interestingly, a decline in nHb to below 9.0 g/dL was significantly related to cerebral infarctions, in-hospital mortality, and poor outcome. These findings are independent of baseline characteristics and adverse clinical events during hospitalization. Previous literature often described anemia as an epiphenomenon of the hemodiluting effects of SAH therapy. Our study provides, for the first time, data on the influence of anemia on poor outcomes in SAH patients, independent of other factors. Our results encourage further prospective evaluations of the value of different transfusion strategies in the functional outcomes of SAH patients.

Supplementary Materials: The following supporting information can be downloaded at: https://www.mdpi.com/article/10.3390/jcm11216258/s1, Table S1: Univariate analysis on the association between different nHb values and potential prognostic factors; Table S2: Multivariate analysis with the M1 (adjusted for baseline characteristics) and M2 models on the association between different nHb values and the major outcome endpoints of the study; Table S3: Analysis of the association between the timing of outcome-relevant nHb <9.0 g/dL and the major study endpoints.

Author Contributions: Conceptualization, M.S. and R.J. methodology, R.J.; formal analysis, R.J.; investigation, M.S. and R.J.; resources, R.J.; data curation, M.S., T.F.D., M.G., L.R., M.C., J.R., M.D.O. and R.J.; writing—original draft preparation, M.S.; writing—review and editing, T.F.D., L.R., M.C., J.R., V.L., M.D.O., P.D., A.-K.U., K.H.W., U.S. and R.J.; visualization, M.S. and R.J.; supervision, R.J.; project administration, M.S.; funding acquisition, M.S. and R.J. All authors have read and agreed to the published version of the manuscript.

Funding: We acknowledge support by the Open Access Publication Fund of the University of Duisburg-Essen.

Institutional Review Board Statement: The study was conducted in accordance with the Declaration of Helsinki. The study was registered in the German trial registry (DRKS, Unique identifier: RKS00008749) and approved by the local ethics committee (Ethik-Kommission, Medizinische Fakultät der Universität Duisburg-Essen, Registration number: 15-6331-BO).

Informed Consent Statement: Informed consent was obtained from all subjects involved in the study.

Data Availability Statement: Data are available and will be provided by the authors upon reasonable request.

Conflicts of Interest: The authors declare no conflict of interest.

Previous Presentation

ePoster Presentation, DGNC 29 May–1 June 2022, Cologne, Germany.

References

1. Kramer, A.H.; Zygun, D.A.; Bleck, T.P.; Dumont, A.S.; Kassell, N.F.; Nathan, B. Relationship between hemoglobin concentrations and outcomes across subgroups of patients with aneurysmal subarachnoid hemorrhage. *Neurocrit Care* **2009**, *10*, 157–165. [CrossRef]
2. Sun, J.; Tan, G.; Xing, W.; He, Z. Optimal hemoglobin concentration in patients with aneurysmal subarachnoid hemorrhage after surgical treatment to prevent symptomatic cerebral vasospasm. *Neuroreport* **2015**, *26*, 263–266. [CrossRef] [PubMed]
3. Naidech, A.M.; Drescher, J.; Ault, M.L.; Shaibani, A.; Batjer, H.H.; Alberts, M.J. Higher hemoglobin is associated with less cerebral infarction, poor outcome, and death after subarachnoid hemorrhage. *Neurosurgery* **2006**, *59*, 775–779. [CrossRef] [PubMed]
4. Ayling, O.G.S.; Ibrahim, G.M.; Alotaibi, N.M.; Gooderham, P.A.; Macdonald, R.L. Anemia After Aneurysmal Subarachnoid Hemorrhage Is Associated With Poor Outcome and Death. *Stroke* **2018**, *49*, 1859–1865. [CrossRef] [PubMed]
5. Bell, D.L.; Kimberly, W.T.; Yoo, A.J.; Leslie-Mazwi, T.M.; Rabinov, J.D.; Bell, J.E.; Mehta, B.P.; Hirsch, J.A. Low neurologic intensive care unit hemoglobin as a predictor for intra-arterial vasospasm therapy and poor discharge modified Rankin Scale in aneurysmal subarachnoid haemorrhage-induced cerebral vasospasm. *J. Neurointerv. Surg.* **2015**, *7*, 438–442. [CrossRef]
6. Naidech, A.M.; Jovanovic, B.; Wartenberg, K.E.; Parra, A.; Ostapkovich, N.; Connolly, E.S.; Mayer, S.A.; Commichau, C. Higher hemoglobin is associated with improved outcome after subarachnoid hemorrhage. *Crit. Care Med.* **2007**, *35*, 2383–2389. [CrossRef]

7. English, S.W.; Chasse, M.; Turgeon, A.F.; Lauzier, F.; Griesdale, D.; Garland, A.; Fergusson, D.; Zarychanski, R.; van Walraven, C.; Montroy, K.; et al. Anemia prevalence and incidence and red blood cell transfusion practices in aneurysmal subarachnoid hemorrhage: Results of a multicenter cohort study. *Crit. Care* **2018**, *22*, 169. [CrossRef]
8. Le Roux, P.D. Participants in the International Multi-disciplinary Consensus Conference on the Critical Care Management of Subarachnoid, H., Anemia and transfusion after subarachnoid hemorrhage. *Neurocrit Care* **2011**, *15*, 342–353. [CrossRef]
9. Jabbarli, R.; Reinhard, M.; Shah, M.; Roelz, R.; Niesen, W.D.; Kaier, K.; Taschner, C.; Weyerbrock, A.; Van Velthoven, V. Early Vasospasm after Aneurysmal Subarachnoid Hemorrhage Predicts the Occurrence and Severity of Symptomatic Vasospasm and Delayed Cerebral Ischemia. *Cerebrovasc. Dis.* **2016**, *41*, 265–272. [CrossRef]
10. Jabbarli, R.; Darkwah Oppong, M.; Roelz, R.; Pierscianek, D.; Shah, M.; Dammann, P.; Scheiwe, C.; Kaier, K.; Wrede, K.H.; Beck, J.; et al. The PRESSURE score to predict decompressive craniectomy after aneurysmal subarachnoid haemorrhage. *Brain Commun.* **2020**, *2*, fcaa134. [CrossRef]
11. Hebert, P.C.; Wells, G.; Blajchman, M.A.; Marshall, J.; Martin, C.; Pagliarello, G.; Tweeddale, M.; Schweitzer, I.; Yetisir, E. A multicenter, randomized, controlled clinical trial of transfusion requirements in critical care. Transfusion Requirements in Critical Care Investigators, Canadian Critical Care Trials Group. *N. Engl. J. Med.* **1999**, *340*, 409–417. [CrossRef] [PubMed]
12. Teasdale, G.M.; Drake, C.G.; Hunt, W.; Kassell, N.; Sano, K.; Pertuiset, B.; De Villiers, J.C. A universal subarachnoid hemorrhage scale: Report of a committee of the World Federation of Neurosurgical Societies. *J. Neurol. Neurosurg. Psychiatry* **1988**, *51*, 1457. [CrossRef] [PubMed]
13. Fisher, C.M.; Kistler, J.P.; Davis, J.M. Relation of cerebral vasospasm to subarachnoid hemorrhage visualized by computerized tomographic scanning. *Neurosurgery* **1980**, *6*, 1–9. [CrossRef] [PubMed]
14. van Swieten, J.C.; Koudstaal, P.J.; Visser, M.C.; Schouten, H.J.; van Gijn, J. Interobserver agreement for the assessment of handicap in stroke patients. *Stroke* **1988**, *19*, 604–607. [CrossRef] [PubMed]
15. Marik, P.E. The risks of blood transfusion in patients with subarachnoid hemorrhage. *Neurocrit Care* **2012**, *16*, 343–345. [CrossRef]
16. Kramer, A.H.; Gurka, M.J.; Nathan, B.; Dumont, A.S.; Kassell, N.F.; Bleck, T.P. Complications associated with anemia and blood transfusion in patients with aneurysmal subarachnoid hemorrhage. *Crit. Care Med.* **2008**, *36*, 2070–2075. [CrossRef]
17. Sampson, T.R.; Dhar, R.; Diringer, M.N. Factors associated with the development of anemia after subarachnoid hemorrhage. *Neurocrit Care* **2010**, *12*, 4–9. [CrossRef]
18. Wartenberg, K.E.; Schmidt, J.M.; Claassen, J.; Temes, R.E.; Frontera, J.A.; Ostapkovich, N.; Parra, A.; Connolly, E.S.; Mayer, S.A. Impact of medical complications on outcome after subarachnoid hemorrhage. *Crit. Care Med.* **2006**, *34*, 617–623. [CrossRef]
19. Festic, E.; Rabinstein, A.A.; Freeman, W.D.; Mauricio, E.A.; Robinson, M.T.; Mandrekar, J.; Zubair, A.C.; Lee, A.S.; Gajic, O. Blood transfusion is an important predictor of hospital mortality among patients with aneurysmal subarachnoid hemorrhage. *Neurocrit Care* **2013**, *18*, 209–215. [CrossRef]
20. Kim, E.; Kim, H.C.; Park, S.Y.; Lim, Y.J.; Ro, S.H.; Cho, W.S.; Jeon, Y.T.; Hwang, J.W.; Park, H.P. Effect of Red Blood Cell Transfusion on Unfavorable Neurologic Outcome and Symptomatic Vasospasm in Patients with Cerebral Aneurysmal Rupture: Old versus Fresh Blood. *World Neurosurg.* **2015**, *84*, 1877–1886. [CrossRef]
21. Smith, M.J.; Le Roux, P.D.; Elliott, J.P.; Winn, H.R. Blood transfusion and increased risk for vasospasm and poor outcome after subarachnoid hemorrhage. *J. Neurosurg.* **2004**, *101*, 1–7. [CrossRef] [PubMed]
22. Broessner, G.; Lackner, P.; Hoefer, C.; Beer, R.; Helbok, R.; Grabmer, C.; Ulmer, H.; Pfausler, B.; Brenneis, C.; Schmutzhard, E. Influence of red blood cell transfusion on mortality and long-term functional outcome in 292 patients with spontaneous subarachnoid hemorrhage. *Crit. Care Med.* **2009**, *37*, 1886–1892. [CrossRef] [PubMed]
23. Kumar, M.A.; Boland, T.A.; Baiou, M.; Moussouttas, M.; Herman, J.H.; Bell, R.D.; Rosenwasser, R.H.; Kasner, S.E.; Dechant, V.E. Red blood cell transfusion increases the risk of thrombotic events in patients with subarachnoid hemorrhage. *Neurocrit Care* **2014**, *20*, 84–90. [CrossRef] [PubMed]
24. Kramer, A.H.; Diringer, M.N.; Suarez, J.I.; Naidech, A.M.; Macdonald, L.R.; Le Roux, P.D. Red blood cell transfusion in patients with subarachnoid hemorrhage: A multidisciplinary North American survey. *Crit. Care* **2011**, *15*, R30. [CrossRef] [PubMed]
25. Luostarinen, T.; Lehto, H.; Skrifvars, M.B.; Kivisaari, R.; Niemela, M.; Hernesniemi, J.; Randell, T.; Niemi, T. Transfusion Frequency of Red Blood Cells, Fresh Frozen Plasma, and Platelets During Ruptured Cerebral Aneurysm Surgery. *World Neurosurg.* **2015**, *84*, 446–450. [CrossRef]
26. Kumar, M.A.; Levine, J.; Faerber, J.; Elliott, J.P.; Winn, H.R.; Doerfler, S.; Le Roux, P. The Effects of Red Blood Cell Transfusion on Functional Outcome after Aneurysmal Subarachnoid Hemorrhage. *World Neurosurg.* **2017**, *108*, 807–816. [CrossRef]
27. Springer, M.V.; Schmidt, J.M.; Wartenberg, K.E.; Frontera, J.A.; Badjatia, N.; Mayer, S.A. Predictors of global cognitive impairment 1 year after subarachnoid hemorrhage. *Neurosurgery* **2009**, *65*, 1043–1050. [CrossRef]
28. Stein, M.; Brokmeier, L.; Herrmann, J.; Scharbrodt, W.; Schreiber, V.; Bender, M.; Oertel, M.F. Mean hemoglobin concentration after acute subarachnoid hemorrhage and the relation to outcome, mortality, vasospasm, and brain infarction. *J. Clin. Neurosci.* **2015**, *22*, 530–534. [CrossRef]
29. Jaja, B.N.R.; Saposnik, G.; Lingsma, H.F.; Macdonald, E.; Thorpe, K.E.; Mamdani, M.; Steyerberg, E.W.; Molyneux, A.; Manoel, A.L.O.; Schatlo, B.; et al. Development and validation of outcome prediction models for aneurysmal subarachnoid haemorrhage: The SAHIT multinational cohort study. *BMJ* **2018**, *360*, j5745. [CrossRef]
30. Shalev, H.; Kapelushnik, J.; Moser, A.; Knobler, H.; Tamary, H. Hypocholesterolemia in chronic anemias with increased erythropoietic activity. *Am. J. Hematol.* **2007**, *82*, 199–202. [CrossRef]

31. Paul, B.; Wilfred, N.C.; Woodman, R.; Depasquale, C. Prevalence and correlates of anaemia in essential hypertension. *Clin. Exp. Pharmacol. Physiol.* **2008**, *35*, 1461–1464. [CrossRef] [PubMed]
32. Sonnweber, T.; Pizzini, A.; Tancevski, I.; Loffler-Ragg, J.; Weiss, G. Anaemia, iron homeostasis and pulmonary hypertension: A review. *Intern. Emerg. Med* **2020**, *15*, 573–585. [CrossRef] [PubMed]
33. Singh, D.K.; Winocour, P.; Farrington, K. Erythropoietic stress and anemia in diabetes mellitus. *Nat. Rev. Endocrinol.* **2009**, *5*, 204–210. [CrossRef] [PubMed]
34. Wartenberg, K.E.; Mayer, S.A. Medical complications after subarachnoid hemorrhage. *Neurosurg. Clin. N Am.* **2010**, *21*, 325–338. [CrossRef] [PubMed]
35. Macdonald, R.L.; Kassell, N.F.; Mayer, S.; Ruefenacht, D.; Schmiedek, P.; Weidauer, S.; Frey, A.; Roux, S.; Pasqualin, A.; Investigators, C. Clazosentan to overcome neurological ischemia and infarction occurring after subarachnoid hemorrhage (CONSCIOUS-1): Randomized, double-blind, placebo-controlled phase 2 dose-finding trial. *Stroke* **2008**, *39*, 3015–3021. [CrossRef]
36. Rumalla, K.; Lin, M.; Ding, L.; Gaddis, M.; Giannotta, S.L.; Attenello, F.J.; Mack, W.J. Risk Factors for Cerebral Vasospasm in Aneurysmal Subarachnoid Hemorrhage: A Population-Based Study of 8346 Patients. *World Neurosurg.* **2021**, *145*, e233–e241. [CrossRef]
37. Scharte, M.; Fink, M.P. Red blood cell physiology in critical illness. *Crit. Care Med.* **2003**, *31* (Suppl. 12), S651–S657. [CrossRef]
38. Darveau, M.; Denault, A.Y.; Blais, N.; Notebaert, E. Bench-to-bedside review: Iron metabolism in critically ill patients. *Crit. Care* **2004**, *8*, 356–362. [CrossRef]
39. Kumar, M.A. Red blood cell transfusion in the neurological ICU. *Neurotherapeutics* **2012**, *9*, 56–64. [CrossRef]

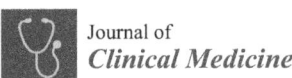

Article

Morphometric Study of the Initial Ventricular Indices to Predict the Complications and Outcome of Aneurysmal Subarachnoid Hemorrhage

Maryam Said [1,2,*], Meltem Gümüs [1,2], Jan Rodemerk [1,2], Mehdi Chihi [1,2], Laurèl Rauschenbach [1,2], Thiemo F. Dinger [1,2], Marvin Darkwah Oppong [1,2], Yahya Ahmadipour [1,2], Philipp Dammann [1,2], Karsten H. Wrede [1,2], Ulrich Sure [1,2] and Ramazan Jabbarli [1,2]

1 Department of Neurosurgery and Spine Surgery, University Hospital of Essen, 45147 Essen, Germany
2 Center for Translational Neuro & Behavioral Sciences (C-TNBS), University Duisburg Essen, 45127 Essen, Germany
* Correspondence: maryam.said@uk-essen.de

Abstract: Objective: Acute hydrocephalus is a common complication in patients with aneurysmal subarachnoid hemorrhage (SAH). Several ventricular indices have been introduced to enable measurements of ventricular morphology. Previously, researchers have showed their diagnostic value for various neurological disorders. In this study, we evaluated the association between ventricular indices and the clinical course, occurrence of complications and outcome of SAH. Methods: A total of 745 SAH patients with available early admission computed tomography scans were included in the analyses. Six ventricular indices (bifrontal, bicaudate, ventricular and third ventricle ratios and Evans' and Huckman's indices) were measured. Primary endpoints included the occurrence of cerebral infarctions, in-hospital mortality and a poor outcome at 6 months. Secondary endpoints included different adverse events in the course of SAH. Clinically relevant cut-offs for the indices were determined using receiver operating curves. Univariate analyses were performed. Multivariate analyses were conducted on significant findings in a stepwise backward regression model. Results: The higher the values of the ventricular indices were and the older the patient was, the higher the WFNS and Fisher's scores were, and the lower the SEBES score was at admission. Patients with larger ventricles showed a shorter duration of intracranial pressure increase > 20 mmHg and required decompressive craniectomy less frequently. Ventricular indices were independently associated with the parameters of inflammatory response after SAH (C-reactive protein in serum and interleukin-6 in cerebrospinal fluid and fever). Finally, there were independent correlations between larger ventricles and all the primary endpoints. Conclusions: The lower risk of intracranial pressure increase and absence of an association with vasospasm or systemic infections during SAH, and the poorer outcome in individuals with larger ventricles might be related to a more pronounced neuroinflammatory response after aneurysmal bleeding. These observations might be helpful in the development of specific medical and surgical treatment strategies for SAH patients depending on the initial ventricle measurements.

Keywords: subarachnoid hemorrhage; ventricular measurements; inflammation; marker; decompressive craniectomy

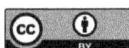

1. Introduction

Subarachnoid hemorrhage (SAH) after an intracranial aneurysm rupture is known to have several severe complications. Acute hydrocephalus in SAH is a very frequent occurring phenomenon, with reported rates of up to 97% [1]. Ventricular morphology, and especially its pathological enlargement, have been a subject of interest for a long time. Anatomical studies on the brain have been conducted since ancient times, and in around the 1500 s, Leonardo da Vinci managed to make a cast out of the ventricular system of an ox [2]. Over time, several animal and human cadaver studies have been conducted on the brain with descriptions of ventricular morphology [3]. The introduction of radiographic imaging immensely aided research on the ventricular system. Ventricular enlargement on a pneumocephalogram was described by Evans in 1942 [4]. The simple index measurement he presented, consisting of the ratio of the maximal diameter of the frontal horns to the internal diameter of the cranial vault, is currently still in use. Since then, several other ventricular measurements have been introduced. Correlations between these measurements and different diseases, such as normal pressure hydrocephalus [5], Morbus Alzheimer [6] and schizophrenia [7], have been described. Ventricular measurements have been incorporated in the guideline for normal pressure hydrocephalus as a diagnostic tool [5]. This illustrates the usefulness ventricular measurements can provide in clinical practice. With the frequent occurrence of acute hydrocephalus in SAH, ventricular measurements may contribute to our advanced understanding of this complicated disease. Previously, it has been shown that in SAH patients with acute hydrocephalus, the cerebral blood flow is reduced, especially in the periventricular regions [8]. Additionally, a correlation between a poor functional outcome after SAH and acute hydrocephalus has been reported [9].

Quantifying this acute hydrocephalus could aid in the prediction of other SAH complications and the final outcome. The aim of our study was to evaluate the association between ventricular indices and the clinical course, occurrence of complications and outcome of SAH by using morphometric data of several ventricular indices.

2. Methods

2.1. Patient Population

For our retrospective cohort study, all consecutive SAH patients that were treated at our institution between January 2003 and June 2016 and were eligible were included. Patients were considered to be eligible when they: (1) were above 18 years of age and (2) had an available pre-treatment computer tomography (CT) scan < 48 h after the aneurysm rupture, allowing the measurement of several ventricular indices. Exclusion criteria were: (1) no SAH treatment received by the patient; (2) no available CT scan or a scan > 48 h after ictus. Our study is imbedded in the clinical trial registered at the German trial registry (DRKS, Unique identifier: RKS00008749). The study was approved by the local ethics committee (Ethik-Kommission, Medizinische Fakultät der Universität Duisburg-Essen, Registration number: 15-6331-BO).

2.2. SAH Management

All patients with SAH who presented at our facility were admitted to the neurosurgical intensive care unit. Rupture of an intracranial aneurysm was confirmed in digital subtraction angiography (DSA), and aneurysms were usually treated within 24 h either by microsurgical clipping or endovascular coiling. In our previous works, our protocol for post-interventional management at the intensive care unit was described [10–12]. In summary, the conservative treatment is composed of maintenance of the mean arterial pressure > 70 mmHg, oral nimodipine for the first 21 days after ictus and consistent normovolemia. External ventricular drainage (EVD) was placed in case of acute hydrocephalus. In case of pathologically increased intracranial pressure (ICP) > 20 mmHg, conservative treatment was initiated, consisting of deep sedation, forced cerebrospinal fluid (CSF) drainage and osmotherapy. As previously described [12], SAH patients with: (a) clinical, intraoperative and/or radiographic signs of intracranial hypertension at admission, and (b) ICP increase in the course of SAH refractory-to-maximal conservative treatment underwent primary and secondary decompressive craniectomy (DC), respectively. Vasospasm management consisted of a daily neurological examination and transcranial Doppler (TCD) sonography, with the endovascular treatment of SAH patients with symptomatic cerebral vasospasm [11]. Laboratory tests of blood and CSF were performed routinely at admission and three times per week, with additional tests performed if they were clinically indicated. CT scans were conducted in case of any neurological deterioration after surgical procedures and around the placement of a permanent CSF diversion.

2.3. Data Management

All available pre-treatment CT scans after admission were reviewed by the first author (M.S.), who was blinded at this time to clinical information. Measurements of the ventricular indices were conducted as previously described. This concerned the bifrontal, bicaudate, ventricular and third ventricle ratios, as well as Evans' and Huckman's indices [3,4,13–16]. A graphical overview of the exact measurements was presented in our previous work (see Supplementary Materials Figure S1).

Furthermore, various demographic (age and sex), clinical (World Federation of Neurosurgical Societies (WFNS) scale [17] at admission and treatment modality), laboratory and radiographic (presence of intraventricular hemorrhage, Fisher's scale [18] and Subarachnoid Early Brain Edema Score (SEBES) [19] at admission) data of patient and SAH characteristics, complications during SAH and outcomes were collected from the institutional aneurysm database. For the assessment of the inflammatory status during SAH, the following laboratory parameters were included (admission and 14 days mean values): white blood cells (leukocytes) and c-reactive protein (CRP) in blood and interleukin-6 (IL-6) in CSF. The clinical/adverse events also recorded for further analysis were: aneurysm rebleeding before treatment, early angiographic vasospasm (documented within 72 h after ictus), occurrence and duration of cerebral vasospasm (s) in TCD (mean flow velocities > 120 cm/s), development of delayed ischemic neurological deficit (DIND), endovascular treatment for vasospasm, epileptic seizures, new cerebral infarction (s) in follow-up CT scans, occurrence of a fever (body temperature > 38.0° at admission and during SAH), duration of ICP increase, need for DC, duration of mechanical ventilation (including the duration of sedation for mechanical ventilation), development of meningitis, systemic infections, acute coronary syndrome and acute renal failure during SAH. For the assessment of the functional outcome of SAH, the rates of in-hospital mortality and unfavorable outcome at 6 months after SAH (defined as modified Rankin Scale > 3 [20]) were included in the analysis.

2.4. Study Endpoints and Statistical Analyses

We aimed to predict the correlation between ventricular morphology and the occurrence of complications in the course of SAH and its final outcome by using measurements of the above-mentioned indices. Our main study endpoints were cerebral infarction, in-hospital mortality and an unfavorable outcome at 6 months. Secondary endpoints included the associations between ventricular indices and the occurrence of the above-mentioned adverse events in the clinical course. The predictive value of ventricular measurements of chronic hydrocephalus and shunt dependency after SAH was analyzed elsewhere.

First, the ventricular indices were evaluated as continuous variables in an explorative manner using the Pearson correlation and the Spearman's rank tests, as appropriate. For further univariate and multivariate analyses, all ventricular indices were dichotomized at the cut-offs defined using the area under the curve (AUC) on the receiver operating characteristic (ROC) analyses for prediction of the primary study endpoints. Thereafter, univariate analyses for correlations between the dichotomized ventricular indices and primary and secondary study endpoints were performed. For categorical variables, the Chi-square test (χ^2 test) or Fisher's exact test, as appropriate, was used. For continuous variables, Student's *t*-test (for normally distributed data) or Mann–Whitney U test (for non-normally distributed data) was applied. Then, multivariate analysis was performed on the significant findings in order to confirm the independent association. Four baseline parameters associated with ventricular indices—age, SEBES, WFNS and Fisher's scores at admission—were included as obligatory components of the multivariate models. Furthermore, the significant ventricular indices were included in a stepwise backward regression model. The associations between ventricular morphology and the burden of ICP increase after SAH were additionally analyzed using Kaplan–Meier survival plots, and the construction of a novel prediction score was achieved using the results of the multivariate analysis. Data analysis was performed using SPSS statistical software (version 25, SPSS Inc., IBM Company, Chicago, IL, USA). Correlations with a *p*-value of <0.05 were considered to be statistically significant.

3. Results

A total of 745 SAH patients in the above-mentioned study period were eligible for our study, and thus, were included in the final cohort. We provide an overview of major demographic, clinical and radiographic characteristics in Table 1.

Table 1. Major demographic, clinical and radiographic characteristics of the final cohort.

Parameter	Number of Cases (% *) or Mean (±SD)
Ventricular measurements	
Bifrontal ratio: A/a	0.339 (±0.057)
Bicaudate ratio: B/b	0.166 (±0.081)
Ventricular ratio: B/A	0.517 (±0.214)
Third ventricle ratio: C/c	0.062 (±0.046)
Evans' index: A/D	0.275 (±0.046)
Huckman's index: A + B (cm)	5.419 (±1.244)
Demographic characteristics	
Age (years)	54.7 (±13.9)
Sex (female)	497 (66.7%)
SAH characteristics	
WFNS (grade 4–5)	360 (48.3%)
SEBES (grade 3–4)	386 (52.1%)
Fisher's scale (grade 3–4)	638 (90.1%)
Clipping	302 (40.5%)
Presence of IVH	390 (52.4%)
Acute hydrocephalus	570 (76.5%)
Neurologic complications during SAH	
Aneurysm rebleeding	49 (6.6%)
DIND	193 (31.3%)
Pathologic ICP increase	368 (49.9%)
Decompressive craniectomy	228 (30.6%)
TCD vasospasm	340 (53.0%)
Early angiographic vasospasms (within 72 h)	57 (9.7%)
Endovascular treatment of vasospasm	171 (23.0%)
Epileptic seizures	68 (9.1%)
Systemic complications during SAH	
Systemic infections	310 (46.3%)
Acute coronary syndrome	20 (3.1%)
Acute kidney failure	9 (1.4%)
Primary study endpoints	
Cerebral infarction (s)	380 (51.4%)
In-hospital mortality	159 (21.3%)
Unfavorable outcome at 6 months (mRS > 3)	296 (42.9%)

Abbreviations: A = maximum width between the two frontal horns; a = internal width of the vault at level of A, B = minimum width of the ventricles between caudate nuclei; b = internal width of the vault at level of B, C = greatest width of the third ventricle; c = internal width of the vault at level of C, D = maximum internal width of the vault. SD = standard deviation; IVH = intraventricular hemorrhage; DIND = delayed ischemic neurological deficit; TCD = transcranial Doppler sonography; SEBES = subarachnoid hemorrhage early brain edema score; WFNS = world federation of neurosurgical societies; DCI = delayed cerebral ischemia; mRS = modified Rankin scale. * Percentages were calculated using the cases with known values.

Initial explorative analyses revealed an association between the ventricular indices as continuous variables, and several recorded parameters (see Supplementary Materials Table S1) showed significant results for patients' demographic characteristics, initial SAH severity and different secondary complications, as well as the primary study endpoints. On the whole, the larger the ventricles at admission were, the poorer the patient's functional outcome was. SAH patients with larger ventricles were more likely to be of older age and present with increased SAH severity (higher WFNS, SEBES and Fisher's grades), but they were at a lower risk of ICP- and vasospasm-related complications during SAH.

For further analyses, clinically relevant cut-offs for the ventricular indices were defined using ROC analyses: bifrontal ratio ≥ 0.337; bicaudate ratio ≥ 0.175; Evans' index ≥ 0.281; ventricular ratio ≥ 0.559; Huckman's index ≥ 5.48; third ventricle ratio ≥ 0.053 (see Supplementary Materials Table S2). Univariate analyses of the dichotomized ventricular indices and the primary/secondary endpoint events are provided in Supplementary Materials Tables S3 and S4.

Finally, all the primary study endpoints and significant adverse events from the univariate analyses were tested by multivariate analysis, which was adjusted for patients' age and initial SAH severity (Table 2). These analyses confirmed an independent association between larger ventricles with a risk of cerebral infarction (ventricular ratio ≥ 0.559: adjusted odds ratio (aOR) = 1.54, p = 0.017), in-hospital mortality (bicaudate ratio ≥ 0.175; aOR = 1.61; p = 0.025) and unfavorable outcome at 6 months (Evans' index ≥ 0.281: aOR = 1.67, p = 0.017; ventricular ratio ≥0.559: aOR = 1.73, p = 0.013).

Table 2. Multivariate analysis for the predictors of the primary study endpoints (cerebral infarction, in-hospital mortality and unfavorable outcome at 6 months after SAH). The model obligatory includes the major baseline confounders (age, WFNS, Fisher's and SEBES grades) displayed as ventricular indices in the backward regression model. Cut-offs of ventricular indices, determined by the AUC according to ROC analyses, were used. For all analyses, only the last steps were included.

Ventricular Ratio/Index	aOR (95% CI)	p-Value
Cerebral infarction		
Age >55 years	1.39 (0.97–1.99)	0.073
WFNS grade 4–5	**2.57 (1.82–3.62)**	**<0.0001**
SEBES 3–4	**1.61 (1.13–2.28)**	**0.008**
Fisher's grade 3–4	1.50 (0.84–2.69)	0.174
Ventricular ratio ≥0.559	**1.54 (1.07–2.19)**	**0.017**
In-hospital mortality		
Age >55 years	**1.81 (1.17–2.79)**	**0.007**
WFNS grade 4–5	**3.57 (2.28–5.58)**	**<0.0001**
SEBES 3–4	1.49 (0.96–2.31)	0.074
Fisher's grade 3–4	4.12 (0.96–17.67)	0.057
Bicaudate ratio ≥0.175	**1.61 (1.06–2.44)**	**0.025**
Unfavorable outcome at 6 months after SAH *		
Age >55 years	**2.75 (1.78–4.23)**	**<0.0001**
WFNS grade 4–5	**7.03 (4.69–10.56)**	**<0.0001**
SEBES 3–4	**1.73 (1.12–2.69)**	**0.013**
Fisher's grade 3–4	**4.68 (1.57–13.97)**	**0.006**
Evans' index ≥0.281	**1.67 (1.10–2.53)**	**0.017**
Ventricular ratio ≥0.559	**1.73 (1.12–2.65)**	**0.013**

Abbreviations: aOR = adjusted odds ratio; CI = confidence interval; AUC = area under the curve; ROC = receiver operating characteristic. SEBES = subarachnoid hemorrhage early brain edema score; WFNS = world federation of neurosurgical societies. * Defined as modified Rankin scale >3. Significant values are in bold.

Regarding the secondary endpoints of the study, the multivariate analysis also showed an independent association between larger ventricles and a lower ICP burden after SAH: lower risk of ICP increase > 20 mmHg (third ventricle ratio ≥ 0.053: aOR = 0.65, p = 0.017) and the need for DC (ventricular ratio ≥ 0.559: aOR = 0.43, p = 0.001). Figure 1 shows the duration of ICP increase in different SAH subpopulations depending on the values of ventricular indices. In the Kaplan–Meier survival analysis, the ventricular ratio ≥ 0.559 proved to be the best fit for prediction of the need for and timing of DC after SAH (Figure 2). Based on the results of the multivariate analysis for the prediction of DC, we constructed a risk score based on significant parameters and appropriate aOR values. Accordingly, the novel risk score for DC prediction (0–5 points) included the following components: WFNS grade 4–5 (1 point), Fisher's grade 3–4 (2 points), SEBES grade 3–4 (1 point) and the ventricular ratio < 0.559 (1 point, see Table 3). The constructed risk score showed a good diagnostic accuracy for the prediction of DC (AUC = 0.754). With increasing points on this risk score, the patients' need for DC increased in the analyzed cohort (see Figure 3).

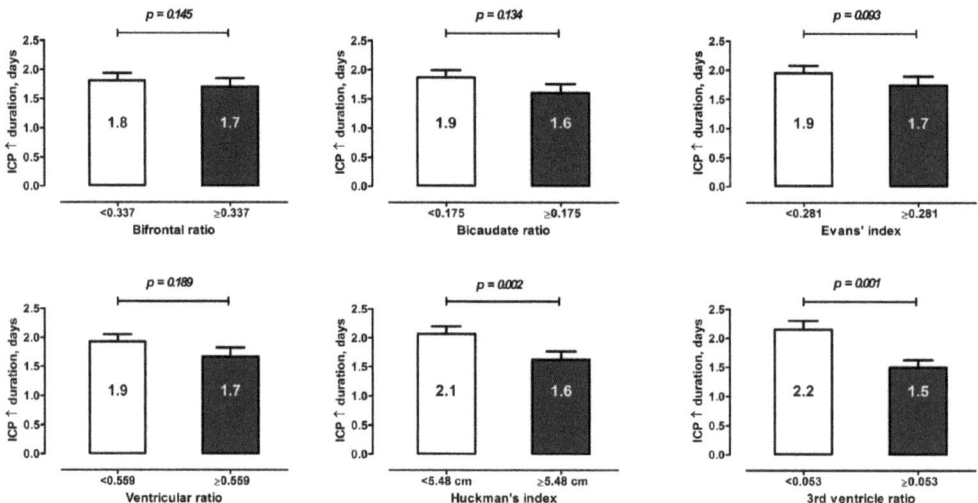

Figure 1. Mean duration of ICP increase after SAH (in days) in different subgroups depending on the values of the ventricular indices. The larger the ventricles are, the shorter the duration of ICP increase > 20 mmHg requiring medical or surgical treatment is.

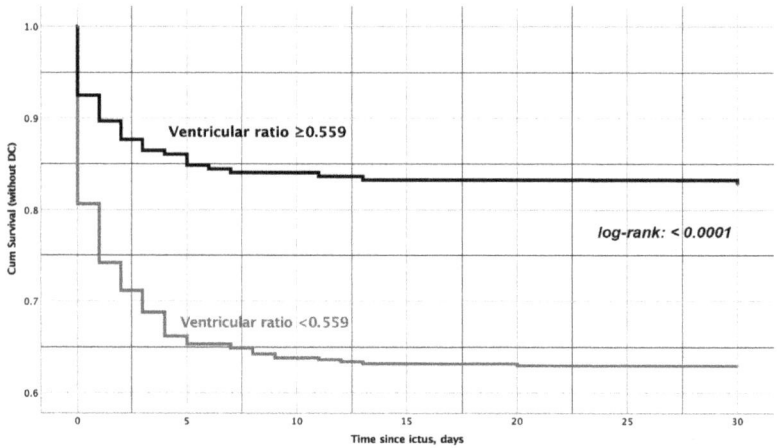

Figure 2. Kaplan–Meier survival plot showing the diagnostic value of the ventricular ratio (with cut-off of 0.559) for predicting the need for DC and its timing. The probability to survive SAH without DC was significantly higher in patients with larger ventricles. SAH patients with smaller ventricles underwent DC more frequently.

Table 3. Components and weights of parameters in the prediction model for decompressive craniectomy.

Parameter	Score Weight
WFNS grade 4–5	1
SEBES 3–4	1
Fisher's grade 3–4	2
Ventricular ratio <0.559	1

Abbreviations: WFNS = world federation of neurosurgical societies; SEBES = subarachnoid early brain edema score.

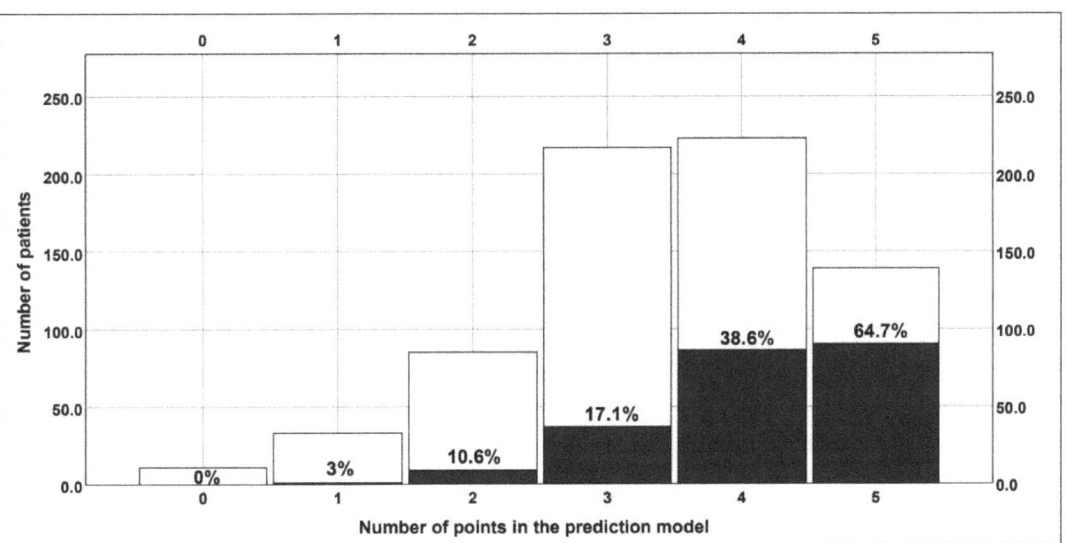

Figure 3. Risk prediction model for the need of DC in SAH patients based on four independent predictors from the multivariate analysis (see Supplementary Materials Table S5): SEBES grade 3–4, ventricular ratio < 0.559, WFNS grade 4–5 and Fisher's grade 3–4. With every point increase in this score, the probability for the need for DC increases. Grey = percentage of patients in need of DC out of all patients with the same score (white ones).

From the remaining multivariate analyses, the ventricular indices showed no link between the risk of aneurysm rebleeding, cerebral vasospasm on TCD or DSA and the occurrence of systemic complications during SAH, such as systemic infections, acute coronary syndrome and acute renal failure. At the same time, larger ventricles were significantly and independently associated with several parameters of highly inflammatory responses at the beginning and during the course of SAH, including CRP in the blood (Evans' index $\geq$ 0.281: aOR = 1.55, p = 0.011; ventricular ratio $\geq$ 0.559: aOR = 1.49, p = 0.031) and IL-6 in CSF (third ventricle ratio $\geq$ 0.053: aOR = 1.69, p = 0.047), as well the duration of a fever (Evans' index $\geq$ 0.281: aOR = 1.55, p = 0.012, see also Figure 4). Of note, the association between the third ventricle ratio and IL6 course in CSF was present, independent of the occurrence of bacterial meningitis during SAH.

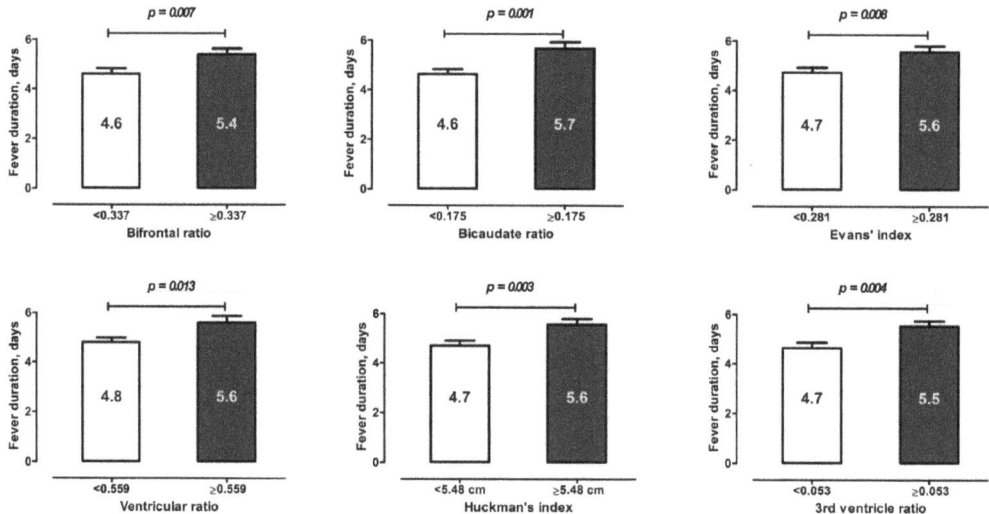

Figure 4. Mean duration of fever after SAH (in days) in different subgroups depending on the values of the ventricular indices. Larger ventricles are significantly and independently associated with a longer duration of fever.

4. Discussion

To our knowledge, this is the first study to evaluate the value of ventricular indices for the prediction of different complications and the outcome of SAH. We showed that the initial ventricular morphology after the bleeding event is strongly associated with the functional outcome of SAH. At the same time, patients with larger ventricles showed fewer complications related to the pathological ICP increase and no link with cerebral vasospasm, but a remarkable inflammatory response at the beginning and during the course of SAH.

Aneurysm rupture leads to a cascade of pathophysiologic processes at the molecular and cellular levels, such as cortical spreading depolarization, microcirculatory failure, cytotoxic and vasogenic edema, oxidative stress, microthrombosis and apoptosis, which later transform into clinically evident complications, such as ICP increase and the development of delayed cerebral ischemia (DCI) [21]. The occurrence and severity of these outcome-relevant pathophysiologic processes depends, at least partially, on the extent of the local and systemic inflammatory responses to the aneurysmal bleeding and the subsequent early brain injury [22]. Neuroinflammation within the brain is driven by inflammatory cells, both those that are locally present and circulating peripherally, and mediated by reactive oxygen species, cytokines, chemokines and other messenger molecules [23–25].

The first studies analyzing inflammation after SAH have attempted to identify a link between inflammation and the risk of cerebral vasospasm [26,27]. Recent studies also identified a higher risk of DCI with increasing inflammatory response after SAH [28,29]. However, this association is probably due to the involvement of inflammatory mediators in the coagulation cascades, resulting in microthrombosis and microcirculatory disturbances, and accordingly, a higher risk of DCI, rather being than related to the vasospasm of large intracranial vessels [30]. Fittingly, several studies have shown a robust association between the level of inflammatory markers in peripheral blood and the occurrence of cerebral infarcts and a poor outcome after SAH [31]. Therefore, the inhibition of inflammation after SAH with medical agents might present a therapeutic target for the prevention of a secondary brain injury after SAH. There are data from small cohort studies that show the positive clinical effect of glucocorticoid treatment in SAH patients [32–34]. This effect might show up in the early phase of SAH by the suppression of microenvironmental and systemic cytokine releases involved in different pathways of an early brain injury [35,36]. Moreover, the increased downregulation of inflammatory cytokines by continuous dexamethasone administration can also contribute to the prevention of secondary SAH complications such as DCI. To assess the above-mentioned results and other potential mechanisms of the glucocorticoids effect, the organizers of a multi-center prospective trial analyzing the effect of treatment with dexamethasone on the SAH outcome are currently recruiting patients in Germany [29].

In the context of the above-described evidence on the impact of inflammation on SAH, the early identification of individuals with a pronounced inflammatory response to SAH is of paramount clinical importance. So, the timely and correct selection of SAH individuals who would benefit from an anti-inflammatory treatment would help to improve the outcome of affected patients, without the overtreatment of cases not showing more extensive inflammation. This circumstance underlines the relevance of our study results. We showed the association between larger ventricles at admission and a higher expression of inflammatory parameters in the blood and CSF, as well as longer duration of a fever during SAH. The exact pathophysiologic background of the link between initial ventricle enlargement and inflammatory response after SAH is unclear. Previous animal studies reported that the association between posthemorrhagic hydrocephalus and elevated inflammation might be conditioned, at least in part, by elevated levels of activity of choroid plexus membrane transporters involved in CSF secretion [37]. According to our results, the ventricle morphology at admission seems to be an early and reliable radiographic marker of the severity of SAH-induced inflammation. The fact that there was no association between the ventricle measurements and systemic infections might indicate the specificity of ventricular indices for inflammatory processes within the injured brain. The absence of a link between larger ventricles and a high risk of ICP- and vasospasm-related complications after SAH also accounts for the decisive role of neuroinflammation as the mediator of the observed association between larger ventricles and the poor outcome of SAH in our cohort. Further clinical and experimental studies to confirm our findings are needed.

So far, the role of ventricular morphology for SAH patients has been addressed only with regard to the prediction of shunt dependency in two small SAH cohorts [38,39]. In our study, along with the independent correlation found between the poor functional outcome of SAH and larger ventricles at admission, we also showed an inverse association between ventricle size and the risk of ICP-related complications. In particular, the larger the ventricles are after aneurysm bleeding on admission CT scans, the lower the risk of ICP increase requiring conservative and surgical treatments is. The duration of pathologic ICP increase was also shorter in SAH individuals with larger ventricles. This inverse association of ventricle morphology with documented ICP increases might be explained by the more pronounced ICP-reducing effect of EVD in these individuals, helping to control the ICP without (or at least with less) documentation of a pathologic ICP increase. As result, SAH patients with initially enlarged ventricles required less frequent additional medical or surgical interventions to reduce the ICP increase.

The observed association between ventricle size and the burden of ICP after SAH is also of clinical relevance. In particular, we constructed a risk score for the need of DC after SAH using independent predictors from the multivariate analysis, including ventricle morphology. The presented novel score based on early and easily assessable clinical and radiographic parameters showed a high diagnostic accuracy for the prediction of DC in SAH patients. The timely selection of SAH individuals needing DC might be helpful in their outcome improvement, as it has been shown in a recent study [12]. Prior to clinical application, an external validation of the presented risk score is necessary.

In summary, provided that we obtain confirmation of our findings on the value of ventricle morphology as an early reliable radiographic marker of the post-SAH inflammatory response and the need for DC in future experimental and clinical studies, the measurement of ventricular indices at admission might be included in decision algorithms for SAH patients. In particular, individuals with severe SAH (WFNS grade 4–5 and Fisher's grade 3–4) with ventricular ratio ≥ 0.559 might benefit from anti-inflammatory treatment (e.g., with glucocorticoids), whereas SAH individuals with a narrow ventricle system (ventricular ratio < 0.559) might be more eligible for early DC.

Limitations

The retrospective and monocentric design of our study are its biggest limitations, resulting in a number of potential research biases that cannot be fully ruled out. Therefore, no judgment on a true causal relationship between the significant study results can be made; thus, different hypotheses may be proposed. Although they are currently of rather speculative nature, these hypotheses might become future targets for clinical and experimental research. Nevertheless, our study is based on a large representative SAH cohort. The analyses included different statistical assessments to address the potential confounding effect of other parameters. The findings of our study require validation in future clinical and experimental studies.

5. Conclusions

According to our study results, SAH patients with larger ventricles are at a higher risk of cerebral infarctions, in-hospital mortality and an unfavorable outcome at 6 months after SAH. The absence of a correlation with higher ICP or vasospasm risk values indicates that the observed outcome effect might be related to a more extensive inflammatory response documented in SAH individuals with larger ventricles. Therefore, ventricular indices might be a valuable radiographic marker of post-SAH neuroinflammation, helping to identify the individuals who are more likely to benefit from therapeutic anti-inflammatory measures. The diagnostic value of ventricle morphology for DC prediction might aid the timely selection of SAH patients requiring DC.

Supplementary Materials: The following supporting information can be downloaded at: https://www.mdpi.com/article/10.3390/jcm12072585/s1, Figure S1: Illustration of the ventricular measurements. Table S1: Exploratory analyses based on the bivariate associations between the ventricular indices (as continuous variables) and other parameters included in this study. Table S2: ROC analysis for the association between the ventricular measurements and primary study endpoint (unfavorable outcome at 6 months after SAH defined as modified Rankin scale > 3). Based on the AUC values a clinically relevant cut-off was determined for the ventricular ratios and indices. Table S3: Univariate analysis of the ventricular indices and other categorical variables. Ventricular indices are dichotomized at clinically relevant cut-off values, according to the AUC of the ROC curves. All major endpoint, as well as older age, clipping, severe SEBES, IVH, DC and infectious parameters are significantly correlated to higher ventricular indices. Table S4: Univariate analysis of adverse events. The ventricular indices are dichotomized according to the AUC in the ROC analyses. In all ventricular indices, higher values correspond with longer fever and higher inflammatory parameters in serum and CSF. Table S5: Multivariate analyses of the predictors of the secondary study endpoints using binary logistic regression with obligatory inclusion of major confounders (patients' age and WFNS, Fisher and SEBES grades at admission) enhanced by the ventricle indices included in the stepwise back-ward regression model (only the last steps are shown here). For the multivariate analysis of the predictors of mean 14-days CSF IL-6, bacterial meningitis was included as an additional confounder to the prediction model. The continuous endpoints were dichotomized according to the common reference values or the mean/median values within the analyzed cohort. Only the last step of each multivariate analysis is shown.

Author Contributions: Conceptualization, M.S. and R.J.; methodology, R.J.; software, R.J.; validation, R.J.; formal analysis, R.J.; investigation, M.S. and R.J.; resources, M.S. and R.J.; data curation, M.S., M.G., J.R., M.C., L.R., T.F.D. and M.D.O.; writing—original draft, M.S.; writing—review & editing, M.G., J.R., M.C., L.R., T.F.D., M.D.O., Y.A., P.D., K.H.W., U.S. and R.J.; visualization, R.J.; supervision, R.J.; project administration, M.S. All authors have read and agreed to the published version of the manuscript.

Funding: We acknowledge funding of the APC by the Open Access Foundation of the University Duisburg-Essen. No other funding was received.

Institutional Review Board Statement: The study was approved by the local ethics committee (Ethik-Kommission, Medizinische Fakultät der Universität Duisburg-Essen, Registration number: 15-6331-BO).

Informed Consent Statement: All persons or their relatives gave their informed consent within the written treatment contract signed on admission to our institution.

Data Availability Statement: Data are available upon reasonable request by contacting the first author.

Conflicts of Interest: The authors declare no conflict of interest.

References

1. Erixon, H.O.; Sorteberg, A.; Sorteberg, W.; Eide, P.K. Predictors of shunt dependency after aneurysmal subarachnoid hemorrhage: Results of a single-center clinical trial. *Acta Neurochir.* **2014**, *156*, 2059–2069. [CrossRef]
2. Paluzzi, A.; Belli, A.; Bain, P.; Viva, L. Brain 'imaging' in the Renaissance. *J. R. Soc. Med.* **2007**, *100*, 540–543. [CrossRef]
3. LeMay, M. Radiologic changes of the aging brain and skull. *Am. J. Neuroradiol.* **1984**, *143*, 383–389. [CrossRef] [PubMed]
4. Evans, W.J. An encephalographic ratio for estimating ventricular enlargement and cerebral atrophy. *Arch. Neurol. Psychiatry* **1942**, *47*, 931–937. [CrossRef]
5. Nakajima, M.; Yamada, S.; Miyajima, M.; Ishii, K.; Kuriyama, N.; Kazui, H.; Kanemoto, H.; Suehiro, T.; Yoshiyama, K.; Kameda, M.; et al. Guidelines for Management of Idiopathic Normal Pressure Hydrocephalus (Third Edition): Endorsed by the Japanese Society of Normal Pressure Hydrocephalus. *Neurol. Med. Chir.* **2021**, *61*, 63–97. [CrossRef] [PubMed]
6. Karypidou, E.; Megagiannis, P.; Papaoikonomou, D.; Pelteki, N.; Gkatzima, O.; Tsolaki, M. Callosal Angle and Evans Index predict beta amyloid and tau protein in patients with dementia. *Hell. J. Nucl. Med.* **2019**, *22*, 51–58. [PubMed]
7. Andreasen, N.C.; Olsen, S.A.; Dennert, J.W.; Smith, M.R. Ventricular enlargement in schizophrenia: Relationship to positive and negative symptoms. *Am. J. Psychiatry* **1982**, *139*, 297–302. [CrossRef] [PubMed]
8. van Asch, C.J.; van der Schaaf, I.C.; Rinkel, G.J. Acute hydrocephalus and cerebral perfusion after aneurysmal subarachnoid hemorrhage. *Am. J. Neuroradiol.* **2010**, *31*, 67–70. [CrossRef]
9. Dupont, S.; Rabinstein, A.A. Extent of acute hydrocephalus after subarachnoid hemorrhage as a risk factor for poor functional outcome. *Neurol. Res.* **2013**, *35*, 107–110. [CrossRef]
10. Said, M.; Gumus, M.; Herten, A.; Dinger, T.F.; Chihi, M.; Darkwah Oppong, M.; Deuschl, C.; Wrede, K.H.; Kleinschnitz, C.; Sure, U.; et al. Subarachnoid Hemorrhage Early Brain Edema Score (SEBES) as a radiographic marker of clinically relevant intracranial hypertension and unfavorable outcome after subarachnoid hemorrhage. *Eur. J. Neurol.* **2021**, *28*, 4051–4059. [CrossRef]
11. Darkwah Oppong, M.; Buffen, K.; Pierscianek, D.; Herten, A.; Ahmadipour, Y.; Dammann, P.; Rauschenbach, L.; Forsting, M.; Sure, U.; Jabbarli, R. Secondary hemorrhagic complications in aneurysmal subarachnoid hemorrhage: When the impact hits hard. *J. Neurosurg.* **2019**, *132*, 79–86. [CrossRef] [PubMed]
12. Jabbarli, R.; Oppong, M.D.; Dammann, P.; Wrede, K.H.; El Hindy, N.; Ozkan, N.; Muller, O.; Forsting, M.; Sure, U. Time Is Brain! Analysis of 245 Cases with Decompressive Craniectomy due to Subarachnoid Hemorrhage. *World Neurosurg.* **2017**, *98*, 689–694.e2. [CrossRef] [PubMed]
13. Hahn, F.J.; Rim, K. Frontal ventricular dimensions on normal computed tomography. *Am. J. Roentgenol.* **1976**, *126*, 593–596. [CrossRef]
14. Pelicci, L.J.; Bedrick, A.D.; Cruse, R.P.; Vannucci, R.C. Frontal ventricular dimensions of the brain in infants and children. *Arch. Neurol.* **1979**, *36*, 852–853. [CrossRef]
15. Brinkman, S.D.; Sarwar, M.; Levin, H.S.; Morris, H.H., 3rd. Quantitative indexes of computed tomography in dementia and normal aging. *Radiology* **1981**, *138*, 89–92. [CrossRef]
16. Huckman, M.S.; Fox, J.; Topel, J. The validity of criteria for the evaluation of cerebral atrophy by computed tomography. *Radiology* **1975**, *116*, 85–92. [CrossRef] [PubMed]
17. Teasdale, G.M.; Drake, C.G.; Hunt, W.; Kassell, N.; Sano, K.; Pertuiset, B.; De Villiers, J.C. A universal subarachnoid hemorrhage scale: Report of a committee of the World Federation of Neurosurgical Societies. *J. Neurol. Neurosurg. Psychiatry* **1988**, *51*, 1457. [CrossRef]
18. Fisher, C.M.; Kistler, J.P.; Davis, J.M. Relation of cerebral vasospasm to subarachnoid hemorrhage visualized by computerized tomographic scanning. *Neurosurgery* **1980**, *6*, 1–9. [CrossRef]
19. Ahn, S.H.; Savarraj, J.P.; Pervez, M.; Jones, W.; Park, J.; Jeon, S.B.; Kwon, S.U.; Chang, T.R.; Lee, K.; Kim, D.H.; et al. The Subarachnoid Hemorrhage Early Brain Edema Score Predicts Delayed Cerebral Ischemia and Clinical Outcomes. *Neurosurgery* **2018**, *83*, 137–145. [CrossRef]
20. van Swieten, J.C.; Koudstaal, P.J.; Visser, M.C.; Schouten, H.J.; van Gijn, J. Interobserver agreement for the assessment of handicap in stroke patients. *Stroke* **1988**, *19*, 604–607. [CrossRef]
21. Rass, V.; Helbok, R. Early Brain Injury after Poor-Grade Subarachnoid Hemorrhage. *Curr. Neurol. Neurosci. Rep.* **2019**, *19*, 78. [CrossRef] [PubMed]
22. Schneider, U.C.; Xu, R.; Vajkoczy, P. Inflammatory Events Following Subarachnoid Hemorrhage (SAH). *Curr. Neuropharmacol.* **2018**, *16*, 1385–1395. [CrossRef] [PubMed]

23. DiSabato, D.J.; Quan, N.; Godbout, J.P. Neuroinflammation: The devil is in the details. *J. Neurochem.* **2016**, *139* (Suppl. S2), 136–153. [CrossRef] [PubMed]
24. Gilhus, N.E.; Deuschl, G. Neuroinflammation—A common thread in neurological disorders. *Nat. Rev. Neurol.* **2019**, *15*, 429–430. [CrossRef] [PubMed]
25. Jin, J.; Duan, J.; Du, L.; Xing, W.; Peng, X.; Zhao, Q. Inflammation and immune cell abnormalities in intracranial aneurysm subarachnoid hemorrhage (SAH): Relevant signaling pathways and therapeutic strategies. *Front. Immunol.* **2022**, *13*, 1027756. [CrossRef] [PubMed]
26. Minami, N.; Tani, E.; Maeda, Y.; Yamaura, I.; Fukami, M. Effects of inhibitors of protein kinase C and calpain in experimental delayed cerebral vasospasm. *J. Neurosurg.* **1992**, *76*, 111–118. [CrossRef] [PubMed]
27. Mathiesen, T.; Andersson, B.; Loftenius, A.; von Holst, H. Increased interleukin-6 levels in cerebrospinal fluid following subarachnoid hemorrhage. *J. Neurosurg.* **1993**, *78*, 562–567. [CrossRef]
28. Geraghty, J.R.; Lung, T.J.; Hirsch, Y.; Katz, E.A.; Cheng, T.; Saini, N.S.; Pandey, D.K.; Testai, F.D. Systemic Immune-Inflammation Index Predicts Delayed Cerebral Vasospasm After Aneurysmal Subarachnoid Hemorrhage. *Neurosurgery* **2021**, *89*, 1071–1079. [CrossRef]
29. Guresir, E.; Lampmann, T.; Bele, S.; Czabanka, M.; Czorlich, P.; Gempt, J.; Goldbrunner, R.; Hurth, H.; Hermann, E.; Jabbarli, R.; et al. Fight INflammation to Improve outcome after aneurysmal Subarachnoid HEmorRhage (FINISHER) trial: Study protocol for a randomized controlled trial. *Int. J. Stroke* **2022**, *18*, 17474930221093501. [CrossRef]
30. Monsour, M.; Croci, D.M.; Agazzi, S. Microclots in subarachnoid hemorrhage: An underestimated factor in delayed cerebral ischemia? *Clin. Neurol. Neurosurg.* **2022**, *219*, 107330. [CrossRef]
31. Gusdon, A.M.; Savarraj, J.P.J.; Shihabeddin, E.; Paz, A.; Assing, A.; Ko, S.B.; McCullough, L.D.; Choi, H.A. Time Course of Peripheral Leukocytosis and Clinical Outcomes After Aneurysmal Subarachnoid Hemorrhage. *Front. Neurol.* **2021**, *12*, 694996. [CrossRef] [PubMed]
32. Gomis, P.; Graftieaux, J.P.; Sercombe, R.; Hettler, D.; Scherpereel, B.; Rousseaux, P. Randomized, double-blind, placebo-controlled, pilot trial of high-dose methylprednisolone in aneurysmal subarachnoid hemorrhage. *J. Neurosurg.* **2010**, *112*, 681–688. [CrossRef] [PubMed]
33. Czorlich, P.; Sauvigny, T.; Ricklefs, F.; Abboud, T.; Nierhaus, A.; Vettorazzi, E.; Reuter, D.A.; Regelsberger, J.; Westphal, M.; Schmidt, N.O. Impact of dexamethasone in patients with aneurysmal subarachnoid haemorrhage. *Eur. J. Neurol.* **2017**, *24*, 645–651. [CrossRef]
34. Mohney, N.; Williamson, C.A.; Rothman, E.; Ball, R.; Sheehan, K.M.; Pandey, A.S.; Fletcher, J.J.; Jacobs, T.L.; Thompson, B.G.; Rajajee, V. A Propensity Score Analysis of the Impact of Dexamethasone Use on Delayed Cerebral Ischemia and Poor Functional Outcomes After Subarachnoid Hemorrhage. *World Neurosurg.* **2018**, *109*, e655–e661. [CrossRef]
35. Heiss, J.D.; Papavassiliou, E.; Merrill, M.J.; Nieman, L.; Knightly, J.J.; Walbridge, S.; Edwards, N.A.; Oldfield, E.H. Mechanism of dexamethasone suppression of brain tumor-associated vascular permeability in rats. Involvement of the glucocorticoid receptor and vascular permeability factor. *J. Clin. Invest.* **1996**, *98*, 1400–1408. [CrossRef]
36. Lauzier, D.C.; Jayaraman, K.; Yuan, J.Y.; Diwan, D.; Vellimana, A.K.; Osbun, J.W.; Chatterjee, A.R.; Athiraman, U.; Dhar, R.; Zipfel, G.J. Early Brain Injury after Subarachnoid Hemorrhage: Incidence and Mechanisms. *Stroke* **2023**. [CrossRef]
37. Lolansen, S.D.; Rostgaard, N.; Barbuskaite, D.; Capion, T.; Olsen, M.H.; Norager, N.H.; Vilhardt, F.; Andreassen, S.N.; Toft-Bertelsen, T.L.; Ye, F.; et al. Posthemorrhagic hydrocephalus associates with elevated inflammation and CSF hypersecretion via activation of choroidal transporters. *Fluids Barriers CNS* **2022**, *19*, 62. [CrossRef]
38. Rubinos, C.; Kwon, S.B.; Megjhani, M.; Terilli, K.; Wong, B.; Cespedes, L.; Ford, J.; Reyes, R.; Kirsch, H.; Alkhachroum, A.; et al. Predicting Shunt Dependency from the Effect of Cerebrospinal Fluid Drainage on Ventricular Size. *Neurocrit. Care* **2022**, *37*, 670–677. [CrossRef] [PubMed]
39. Weigl, C.; Bruendl, E.; Schoedel, P.; Schebesch, K.M.; Brawanski, A.; Kieninger, M.; Bele, S. III. Ventricle diameter increase during ventricular drainage challenge—A predictor of shunt dependency after subarachnoid hemorrhage. *J. Clin. Neurosci.* **2020**, *72*, 198–201. [CrossRef]

Disclaimer/Publisher's Note: The statements, opinions and data contained in all publications are solely those of the individual author(s) and contributor(s) and not of MDPI and/or the editor(s). MDPI and/or the editor(s) disclaim responsibility for any injury to people or property resulting from any ideas, methods, instructions or products referred to in the content.

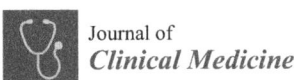

Review

Pathophysiology of Early Brain Injury and Its Association with Delayed Cerebral Ischemia in Aneurysmal Subarachnoid Hemorrhage: A Review of Current Literature

Diana L. Alsbrook [1], Mario Di Napoli [2], Kunal Bhatia [3], Masoom Desai [4], Archana Hinduja [5], Clio A. Rubinos [6], Gelsomina Mansueto [7], Puneetpal Singh [8], Gustavo G. Domeniconi [9], Asad Ikram [10], Sara Y. Sabbagh [4] and Afshin A. Divani [4],*

1. Department of Neurology, University of Tennessee Health Science Center, Memphis, TN 38163, USA
2. Neurological Service, SS Annunziata Hospital, Sulmona, 67039 L'Aquila, Italy
3. Department of Neurology, University of Mississippi Medical Center, Jackson, MS 39216, USA
4. Department of Neurology, University of New Mexico, Albuquerque, NM 87131, USA
5. Department of Neurology, The Ohio State University Wexner Medical Center, Columbus, OH 43210, USA
6. Department of Neurology, University of North Carolina, Chapel Hill, NC 27599, USA
7. Department of Advanced Medical and Surgical Sciences, University of Campania, 80138 Naples, Italy
8. Department of Human Genetics, Punjabi University, Patiala 147002, India
9. Unidad de Cuidados Intensivos, Sanatorio de la Trinidad San Isidro, Buenos Aires 1640, Argentina
10. Stroke Division, Department of Neurology, Beth Israel Deaconess Medical Center, Harvard Medical School, Boston, MA 02115, USA

* Correspondence: adivani@gmail.com

Abstract: *Background:* Delayed cerebral ischemia (DCI) is a common and serious complication of aneurysmal subarachnoid hemorrhage (aSAH). Though many clinical trials have looked at therapies for DCI and vasospasm in aSAH, along with reducing rebleeding risks, none have led to improving outcomes in this patient population. We present an up-to-date review of the pathophysiology of DCI and its association with early brain injury (EBI). *Recent Findings:* Recent studies have demonstrated that EBI, as opposed to delayed brain injury, is the main contributor to downstream pathophysiological mechanisms that play a role in the development of DCI. New predictive models, including advanced monitoring and neuroimaging techniques, can help detect EBI and improve the clinical management of aSAH patients. *Summary:* EBI, the severity of subarachnoid hemorrhage, and physiological/imaging markers can serve as indicators for potential early therapeutics in aSAH. The microcellular milieu and hemodynamic pathomechanisms should remain a focus of researchers and clinicians. With the advancement in understanding the pathophysiology of DCI, we are hopeful that we will make strides toward better outcomes for this unique patient population.

Keywords: aneurysmal subarachnoid hemorrhage; vasospasm; delayed cerebral ischemia; early brain injury; spreading depolarization

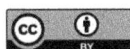

1. Introduction

Aneurysmal subarachnoid hemorrhage (aSAH) (Figure 1) is a devastating stroke subtype with high morbidity and mortality, accounting for approximately 5% of all strokes. A systematic review of population-based studies showed that the crude incidence of aSAH in 2010 in North America was 6.9 per 100,000 person-years with an annual decline of 0.7% since 1955 [1]. However, despite significant advances in diagnosis and management of aSAH, the overall mortality remains high at 35% (range 20–67%) [2,3] and approximately 20% of survivors experience significant morbidity [4], causing a substantial economic and social burden on the patients, families, and healthcare systems [5]. Delayed cerebral ischemia (DCI) is a feared complication of aSAH, increasing the risk of morbidity and mortality, specifically in patients with a severe clinical presentation at ictus and high SAH burden [6,7]. Published data suggests DCI affects approximately 20–40% of aSAH patients and is an independent poor prognostic factor in this population [8–10]. DCI is classically defined as a development of a new neurological deficit(s), impaired consciousness, or infarct on imaging that commences 3 to 4 days after the initial insult and peaks around 7 to 8 days post-bleed [11]. An earlier onset of DCI prior to day 7 has been associated with higher mortality and greater infarct load [12]. Several treatment modalities targeting different pathophysiological pathways causing DCI have been studied. However, there has been minimal change in outcomes due to either DCI prevention or treatment.

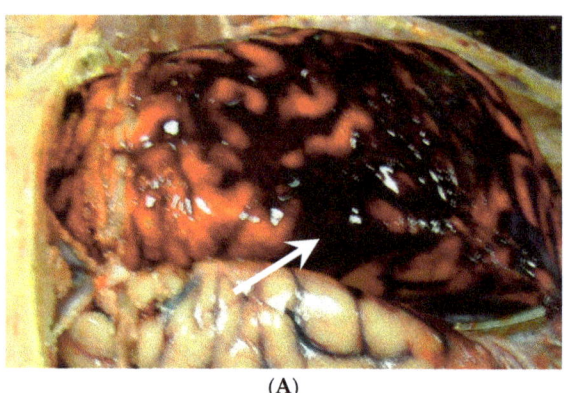 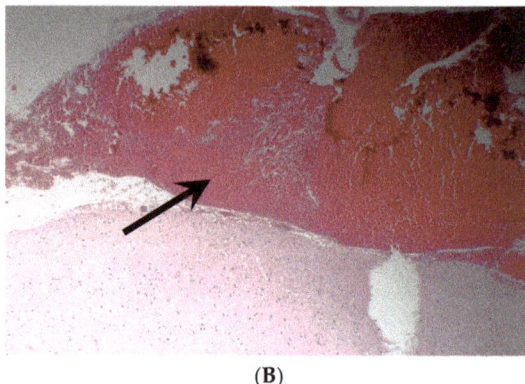

(A) (B)

Figure 1. Subarachnoid hemorrhage. The arrows indicate both macroscopic (**A**) and microscopic (**B**) large bleeding (H&E × 10).

The definition and pathophysiology of this complex and multifactorial process have been debated and studied extensively. In 2007, a study with over 3500 patients [13] evaluated independent variables associated with unfavorable outcomes in aSAH. Authors defined the term "symptomatic vasospasm" as a ≥ 2 point decrease in the Glasgow Coma Scale (GCS) or a ≥ 2 point increase in the motor score of the National Institute of Health Stroke Scale (NIHSS) lasting >8 h, which has since fallen out of favor due to the lack of clear correlation with outcomes. Interestingly, both "symptomatic vasospasm" and cerebral infarction noted on computer tomography (CT) post-operatively showed a significant association with poor functional outcomes at 3 months, with cerebral infarction showing the highest association with unfavorable outcomes (OR = 5.38, $p < 0.0001$) [13]. In 2010, Vergouwen et al. [14] developed a uniform definition of DCI, incorporating clinical deterioration and cerebral infarction as important DCI characteristics that have been well adopted since (see Table 1). Following the definition standardization, in an observational study from Finland that included 340 aSAH patients, 37.1% fulfilled the consensus definition of clinical deterioration secondary to DCI and were strongly associated with poor outcomes at discharge (OR = 2.65, $p < 0.001$) [15]. This has provided an objective, homogenous, and reliable definition of DCI.

For years, large vessel vasospasm was the recognized complication of DCI, leading to the assumption that vasospasm prevention and treatment were paramount in managing aSAH after securing the ruptured aneurysm. However, clazosentan, which was found to treat and reverse vasospasm successfully, failed to improve outcomes. This is possibly because cerebral infarction, secondary to DCI, often occurs in vascular territories outside of the vasoconstricted territories [8,16–18]. Furthermore, DCI has been reported among patients with none or only mild angiographic evidence of vasospasm. Though cerebral vasospasm has been found to occur in 50–70% of aSAH patients, only 20–40% develop DCI [8,13]. Because of this, efforts in the last two decades have been placed on establishing and understanding the pathophysiology of DCI. Hence, the focus has shifted to early brain injury (EBI) and its association with autoregulatory failure, neuroinflammation, and eventually delayed injury (also defined as DCI), with the thought that the treatment of large vessel vasospasms alone might be reactionary and does not address the inciting mechanisms of injury. This review will discuss the current knowledge of pathophysiological mechanisms surrounding EBI and its association with DCI and clinical outcomes after aSAH. In addition, we will discuss the future directions of clinical practice and research to accurately identify various risk factors and strategize therapeutic strategies to improve outcomes in this population.

Table 1. Consensus definition of clinical deterioration and cerebral infarction due to DCI.

Clinical Deterioration Due to DCI	Occurrence of focal neurological impairment (such as hemiparesis, aphasia, apraxia, hemianopia, or neglect), or a decrease of at least 2 points on the GCS (either on the total score or on one of its individual components [eye, motor on either side, verbal]). This should last for at least 1 h, is not apparent immediately after aneurysm occlusion, and cannot be attributed to other causes by means of clinical assessment, CT or MRI scanning of the brain, and appropriate laboratory studies.
Cerebral Infarction Due to DCI	Presence of cerebral infarction on CT or MR scan of the brain within 6 weeks after SAH, or on the latest CT or MR scan made before death within 6 weeks, or proven at autopsy, not present on the CT or MR scan between 24 and 48 h after early aneurysm occlusion, and not attributable to other causes such as surgical clipping or endovascular treatment. Hypodensities on CT imaging resulting from ventricular catheter or intraparenchymal hematoma should not be regarded as cerebral infarctions from DCI.

2. Risk Factors Associated with aSAH and DCI

DCI entails modifiable and non-modifiable pre-morbid risk factors. Though a comprehensive discussion of pre-morbid risk factors is outside this review's scope, Ya et al. [19] noted that smoking was a modifiable risk factor for DCI after aSAH in a meta-analysis. The exact mechanism of this correlation is not well understood, and the role of nicotine is unclear.

Other modifiable and non-modifiable risk factors have been identified in multiple studies. A large multicenter cohort of over 500 patients with aSAH found that female sex, pre-morbid diabetes mellitus, and poor grade aSAH were independent risk factors for DCI [20]. Conversely, Crobeddu et al. [21] reported that older patients (>68 years) with good clinical and radiographic grades were less likely to develop DCI.

Genetic studies have described the role of inheritance patterns in intracranial aneurysm cases, ensuing rupture, and the development of post-rupture complications [22,23]. It has been observed that an individual with a family history of aSAH has a 10% chance of aSAH [24]. A large twins cohort study revealed that the estimated heritability of aSAH is 41% suggesting substantial genetic involvement in its pathogenesis [25]. Candidate gene association studies, meta-analysis, genome-wide association studies (GWAS), and epigenome-wide association studies (EWAS) have exposed several risk variants for unruptured and post-rupture of intracranial aneurysms [26,27]. Interestingly, most (if not all) of the genetic variants observed are unrelated in different studies with discordant inferences. For instance, three meta-analyses have been conducted so far to identify genetic variants responsible for cerebral vasospasm and DCI post-aSAH. The first meta-analysis [28] comprising 16 studies and four genes (endothelial nitric oxide synthase [eNOS], apolipoprotein E [APOE], haptoglobin [Hp], and ryanodine-1 [RYY-1]) demonstrated that carriers of Hp2-2 genotype are at higher risk of developing cerebral vasospasm and DCI. In contrast, another meta-analysis [29] has refuted this claim and showed that Hp2-2 was not associated with either cerebral vasospasm or DCI. The third meta-analysis has suggested that Hp1-2 and Hp1-1 subtypes confer protective effects for cerebral vasospasm and DCI [30]. The possible reasons for such inconsistent results are different sample sizes of the studies deriving variable statistical power, lack of true source of heterogeneity, presence of population stratification, unforeseen epistasis, and miscalculating gene-environmental interactions [31]. A

GWAS examining the gene expression array of blood cells post-aSAH has revealed that the angiogenic and pro-inflammatory gene, neuregulin 1 (NRG1), expresses in patients with DCI and predicts DCI with excellent statistics (AUROC: 0.96) [32]. An EWAS on methylation profiles of patients with DCI has revealed that the hypermethylation of two genes (INSR, CDHR5) at cg00441765 and cg11464053 sites is significantly associated with reduced mRNA expression [33]. Another study has examined DNA methylation vis-à-vis cerebral vasospasm and DCI along with an unfavorable Glasgow Outcome Scale (1–3). The results revealed that methylation site cg25713625 of the STEAP3 gene is significantly associated with unfavorable outcomes and can be used as a therapeutic target for the clinical management of cerebral vasospasm and DCI post-aSAH [34].

Genetic studies are used in clinical practice for decision-making and preventing the worst outcomes of complex diseases [35]. Several genetic variants interact with modifiable risk factors to exhibit heterogeneous effects in complex pathologies such as cerebral vasospasm and DCI. Developing polygenic risk scores (PRS) has ignited a ray of hope that individuals can be risk-stratified on their personalized propensity of the disease [36,37]. A study has utilized the effect estimates for generating weighted PRS (wPRS) by involving 125 intracranial aneurysms and 222 acute ischemic stroke patients in a validation study with 296 matched controls [38]. The risk scoring included 29 GWAS ($p < 5 \times 10^{-8}$) and two already investigated genetic variants ($p < 0.01$), which have shown excellent predictability for intracranial aneurysms (AUROC: 0.95, 95%CI: 0.93–0.97) and acute ischemic stroke (AUROC: 0.842, 95%CI: 0.81–0.88) with a wPRS$_{IA}$ demonstrating a clinical sensitivity of 0.73, specificity of 0.96, and predictability of 0.93 after stratification. This model was able to discriminate intracranial aneurysm patients from controls with an accuracy of 85.5% [38]. Similar future studies will help formulate a quantifiable risk score to improve the clinical decision-making for the prognosis, diagnosis, and therapeutic management in aSAH with formidable complications of cerebral vasospasm and DCI.

3. Pathophysiologic and Hemodynamic Factors Associated with aSAH

Arterial blood enters the subarachnoid space, cisterns, and often into the ventricular system at the time of initial aneurysm rupture (ictus), leading to a higher-pressure system. As the intracranial pressure (ICP) rises, the cerebral perfusion pressure (CPP) is decreased (CPP = MAP–ICP). In a normal physiological condition, a drop in CPP can sustain cerebral blood flow (CBF) to a limited extent prior to autoregulatory dysfunction and failure. However, in a sudden and large increase in ICP, such as in high-grade aSAH, CBF is markedly decreased, leading to the vasodilation of distal cerebral arterioles with the concomitant rise in arterial blood pressure that causes an increase in CBF, further increasing the ICP, until a complete cessation of CBF occurs. This leads to a phenomenon known as "transient global cerebral ischemia" [39]. Early or ictal infarcts can occur during the initial insult where early MRI may be helpful to differentiate this from DCI [11]. Weimer et al. [40] compared the whole brain apparent diffusion coefficient (ADC) on MRI in aSAH patients with controls to quantify the degree of early cytotoxic and vasogenic edema and observed significantly higher ADC values in the aSAH group, providing evidence of early brain edema as a possible mechanism for EBI.

The drop in CPP due to elevated ICP described at ictus is followed closely by a sympathetic catecholamine surge. Injury to the hypothalamus and brainstem, particularly the medulla, due to increased pressure leads to the release of catecholamines mediated by the rostral ventrolateral medulla and the paraventricular nucleus in the hypothalamus [41]. In 1963, Crompton [42] described this phenomenon after aSAH as related to necrosis or hemorrhage of the hypothalamus or damage or vasoconstriction of the arteries that feed it. More recently, this effect was well documented using the diffusion tensor imaging tractography technique showing a decrement in fractional anisotropy and an increase in ADC [43]. The injuries associated with the initial rise in ICP are thought to lead to the accumulation of carbon dioxide and glutamate, which gives rise to reactive astrocytes, and sympathetic activation, followed by secondary activation of the renin-angiotensin-aldosterone system in the kidney [44–46]. This sympathetic reflex has traditionally been recognized as leading to the well-known Cushing response from sympathetic over-excitation due to elevated ICP. The Cushing reflex occurs during prolonged ICP elevation with Lundberg A or plateau waves [47]. However, there has been evidence of an early Cushing-like response, thought to occur in the sudden and early, rather than sustained, rise in ICP after brain injury; this is associated with an intracranial baroreflex and sympatho-excitatory response to raise systemic blood pressure in an attempt to maintain CPP and CBF [48]. Moreover, the catecholamine surge can also lead to endothelin activation, thought to play a role in vasospasm, as well as cytokine release that leads to hyperglycemia, hypokalemia, and leukocytosis. This pathophysiology is the cause of cardiac, lung, renal, and other systemic complications, with a proven dramatic increase in plasma norepinephrine in the setting of cardiac injury in these patients [44,49]. In addition, the insular cortex stimulation with blood spilled due to SAH is realized in paroxysmal sympathetic hyperactivity syndrome [50]. These processes can cause hypotension and hypoxia, which further potentiates brain injury. Though this process starts at the ictus, it continues past the initial injury, causing the process known as EBI.

The prevention of worsening from initial ischemia is of paramount importance post-aSAH. Management of early complications, like rebleeding and hydrocephalus, is an important first step in managing aSAH. Cortical tissue irritation from subarachnoid blood can induce clinical seizures at the onset, most commonly occurring within the first 24 h. This complication occurs in over a quarter of patients, contributing to further increases in cerebral metabolic demand and a secondary increase in ICP due to cerebral blood flow elevations during the ictal period, potentiating ischemia and causing deleterious effects [51]. To manage cerebral autoregulatory failure, bedside blood pressure management is most commonly used, and the maintenance of mean arterial pressure is a mainstay of aSAH management.

In addition to the aforementioned pathophysiological mechanisms, molecular changes contribute to cerebral edema and DCI development. Macrophage migratory inhibitory factor (MIF), a homotrimer protein, has been demonstrated to function as a proinflammatory cytokine capable of activating inflammatory responses in the central nervous system [52,53]. In experimental studies, MIF is released from activated glial cells, which further activate the release of inflammatory mediators from astrocytes leading to brain injury by promoting neuronal cell death [54–56]. In recent studies, serum MIF concentrations have been shown to be associated with severity and long-term outcomes in patients with acute ischemic stroke, traumatic brain injury, and spontaneous intracerebral hemorrhage [57–59]. Similarly, MIF has also been studied as a marker of the severity of brain injury in patients with aSAH. In a prospective study by Chen et al. [53], serum MIF concentrations were found to be significantly higher in patients with aSAH as compared to controls (30.1 ng/mL vs. 7.9 ng/mL; $p < 0.001$). After adjusting for confounding variables (World Federation of Neurosurgical Societies [WFNS] and Fisher scores), serum MIF was identified as an independent predictor for 6-month unfavorable outcomes (Glasgow Outcome Scale Extended, 1–4) in aSAH patients [53]. In another study by Yang et al. [60], higher serum MIF levels were seen in patients who developed DCI as compared to patients without DCI (26.4 [IQR: 22.6–32.4] ng/mL vs. 20.4 [IQR:16.4–24.6] ng/mL, $p < 0.001$). Furthermore, MIF showed a greater discriminatory ability for DCI than the APACHE-II score, C-reactive protein, and interleukin 6 (IL-6) with an AUC of 0.780 (95% CI, 0.710–0.849).

Upregulation of vascular endothelial growth factor and aquaporin-4, increased levels of bradykinin, cytokine release of IL-6, and matrix metalloproteinase-9 are possible targets for treatment, although studies have shown mixed results [51,61]. Drier et al. [62] described that spreading depolarization in the gray matter led to cytotoxic edema, which resulted in ischemia, shown microscopically in Figure 2, leading to neuronal cell death and DCI. Predictive models and prognostication of early edema in aSAH are vast research topics. Wartenberg et al. [63] studied 21 high-grade aSAH patients with early MRI, noting that early ADC diffusion restriction correlates in regions not seen on initial CT. Of those patients,

71% died, and only 12% had a satisfactory outcome. This study proposed that infarcts on CT imaging provided a small picture, and that early MRI could help in noticing and managing early ischemia. In 2018, Ahn et al. [64] evaluated the presence of early edema and noted it as a possible surrogate for EBI and predictor of DCI by designing the Subarachnoid Hemorrhage Early Brain Edema Score (SEBES) that has been recognized as an independent predictor of DCI and is described later in this review. Aside from survival and functional outcome, cerebral edema has also been noted as a predictor of poor cognitive outcomes [61].

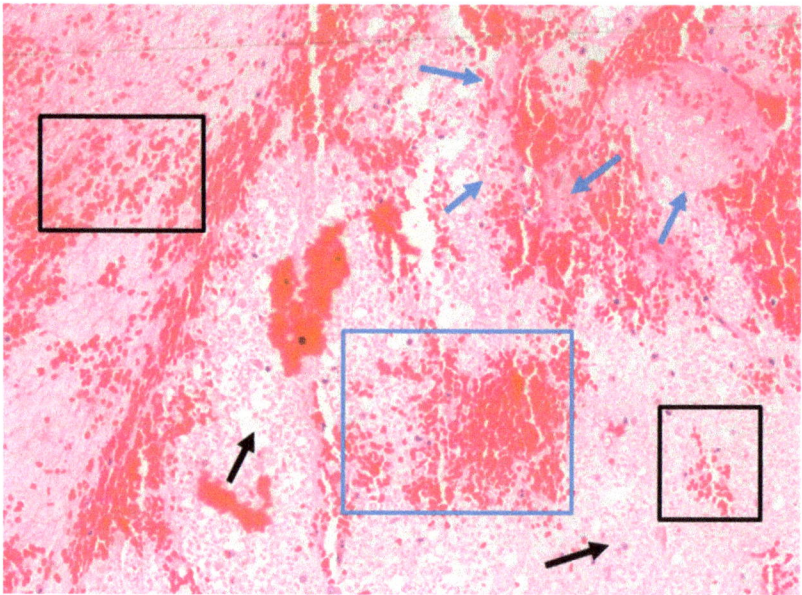

Figure 2. H&E section (×20) showing distribution pattern of erythrocyte extravasations in cerebral ischemia. Intraparenchymal zone in which erythrocyte extravasations are partly diffused (black box), partly wider (blue box), in a context of ischemic necrosis (blue arrow) and edema with aspects of hypoxic cell damage (black arrow).

Early Brain Injury

EBI is believed to occur in the first 72 h following ictus and is a precursor for DCI. Impaired autoregulation is also most prominent in the first 72 h, associated with the increased risk of DCI [65]. The catecholamine surge at ictus continues up to 7 to 10 days post-rupture [44]. As previously mentioned, glutamate accumulation and impaired uptake are part of this process. This causes NMDA receptor activation leading to calcium ion flooding the cell, inducing apoptosis and cell necrosis, as well as the breakdown of the blood-brain barrier (BBB), which all contribute to EBI [65].

Endothelial dysfunction is thought to be a major contributor to vasoconstriction. Oxy- and deoxyhemoglobin damage healthy neurons that secrete neuronal nitric oxide synthase in the brain vessels and parenchyma. The decrease in nitric oxide level needed for vasodilation leads to vasoconstriction. The normal reactionary increase in endothelial nitric oxide synthase is also impaired, which causes continued vasoconstriction until nitric oxide is restored to a normal level [65]. This is also implicated in BBB breakdown due to associated apoptosis and increased permeability, especially in microvessels [65]. Activation of calcium channels and enhanced membrane depolarization are thought to lead to further microvessel spasms [66].

Platelet aggregation is another important contributor to EBI. In animal models, microthrombi from platelet aggregates have been noted as early as 10 min following aSAH.

Punctate infarcts on MRI could be associated with microthrombi and have been shown to predict worse outcomes [67]. Another study that evaluated MRI diffusion restriction in the first four days after poor grade aSAH demonstrated that 86% of patients had diffusion restriction and ADC correlates that were not seen on CT [63].

Cellular loss of ionic gradient leads to cortical spreading depolarization, which is seen as a negative direct current, noting differences in depolarization. Sodium and water enter the depolarized cell, leading to cellular swelling and necrosis. This sustained neuronal depolarization presents as slow-moving and propagating waves, detected using subdural electrodes. In severe cases, this can lead to spreading depolarization-induced spreading depression, which is a decline in the amplitude of the alternating current, or loss of spontaneous electrical activity in the brain [62]. This is associated with injury in a bimodal fashion, with both early and delayed brain injury after aSAH [17,51]. In a recently published pilot clinical trial on depolarizations in ischemia after subarachnoid hemorrhage (DISCHARGE-1) [68], the primary outcome was the peak total depression time from spreading depolarization that was indicative of DCI. The authors hypothesized that a 60-min cutoff of spreading depolarization-induced depression would predict delayed infarction with high sensitivity (>0.6) and specificity (>0.8). However, the study's results revealed that this time interval was too short of reaching the desired specificity of 0.80 (specificity was 0.59), though it reached higher than desired sensitivity (0.76). A 180-min cutoff was found to have lower sensitivity (0.62), but higher specificity (0.83). However, the 60-min cutoff had a higher sensitivity and specificity for predicting DCI than the defined cerebral infarction. In their conclusion, Dreier et al. [68] found that spreading depolarizations were likely an independent marker of brain injury post-aSAH. One episode of spreading depolarization alone was shown to significantly affect the risk of poor outcomes in their studied population. In another study of 19 subjects, Owen et al. [69] reviewed cerebral autoregulation and spreading depolarizations simultaneously through multimodal monitoring. Spreading depolarization was associated with impaired cerebral autoregulation, proposing a negative feedback phenomenon from impaired cerebral autoregulation that leads to decreased CBF and spreading depolarization, leading back to further worsening of cerebral autoregulation. Though there is no consensus, given these findings, it is plausible that cortical spreading depression provokes ischemia. These important studies further support the use of advanced neuromonitoring, especially in high-grade aSAH that also has the potential to provide us with a therapeutic target. Carlson et al. [70] published a pilot study of ketamine to suppress spreading depolarizations in traumatic brain injury and aSAH patients, with a subsequent study to look at an alternative N-methyl-D-aspartate receptor antagonist, memantine, which seems to be a promising alternative [71].

4. Recent Developments

4.1. Subarachnoid Hemorrhage Early Brain Edema Score (SEBES)

The SEBES score is a semi-quantitative CT grading scale that was developed as a novel radiographic marker of EBI, also helpful in predicting DCI and unfavorable outcomes. The score is based on a scale of 0–4 (where 4 presents the worst) and calculated similarly to the Alberta Stroke Program Early CT Score (ASPECTS) [72] in acute ischemic stroke, at two separate slices: Slice 1: the level of the insular cortex, showing the thalamus and basal ganglia, and Slice 2: the level of the centrum semiovale above the level of the lateral ventricle. A point is assigned for each side with effacement of the sulci, at each level, as seen in Figure 3. In a prospective study that included 164 patients, high-grade Hunt and Hess (HH) and higher WFNS grade were identified as predictors of high-grade SEBES score (defined as a score of 3 or 4). After adjusting for covariates, SEBES was identified as an independent predictor of DCI (OR = 2.24, 95% CI: 1.58–3.17) and unfavorable outcome (OR = 3.45, 95% CI: 1.95–6.07) [64]. In another study by Said et al. [73], independent associations were found between higher SEBES scores (3 or 4) and the need for medical management of ICP, decompressive craniectomy, development of cerebral infarction, as well as unfavorable outcomes. In an observational cohort, Rass et al. [74] used the SEBES score repeatedly to follow the course of edema. They concluded that the score could identify patients with delayed resolution of early brain edema. As stated, aggressive control of cerebral edema, and the factors that play a role in the late resolution, should be part of the initial management of these patients using the SEBES score.

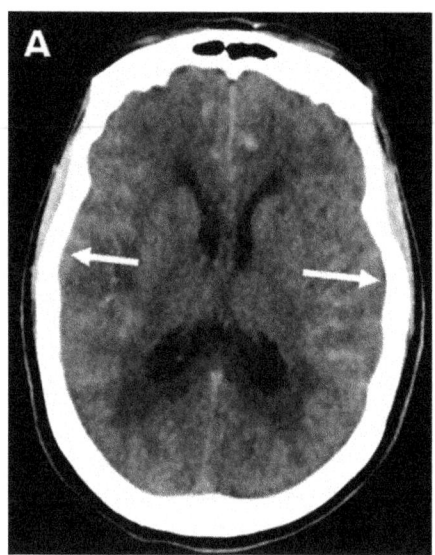 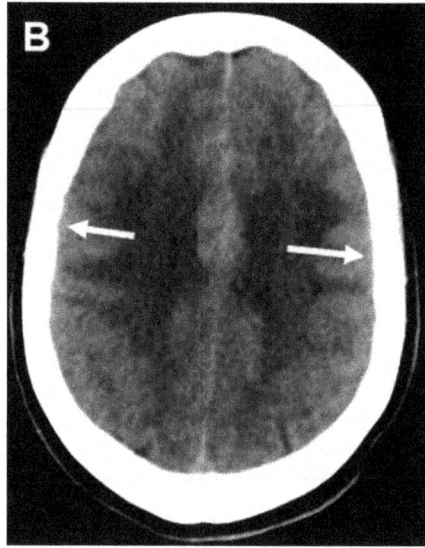

Figure 3. SEBES score calculation from non-contrast CT of the head. (**A**) Slice 1 with 2 points for bilateral effacement of sulci. (**B**) Slice 2 of the same CT with 2 points for bilateral sulcal effacement. The total SEBES score for this scan is 4.

4.2. Volumetric Analysis of Edema

Dhar and his team have recently studied volumetric analysis of global cerebral edema (GCE) as a predictor of poor outcomes after aSAH [75], where the selective sulcal volume (SSV) and the CSF volume above the lateral ventricles were measured using an automated machine learning algorithm and studied as a quantitative biomarker of GCE. In this study, an SSV cutoff below 5 mL accurately identified GCE in patients with aSAH. Furthermore, early SSV (i.e., the lowest SSV within 72 h of ictus) was noted to be an independent predictor of poor outcomes with the strongest impact on the prediction of GCE in younger patients (<70 years old).

4.3. Multimodal Monitoring, Predictive Models, and Diagnosis of Dci

Multimodal monitoring (Table 2) is becoming more widely used in this patient population. It has been shown to aid in detecting DCI, especially in patients with limited reliable secondary brain injury examination [76,77]. Lazaridis's summary of cerebral shock explains different pathophysiologic profiles associated with these monitoring techniques, summarized in Table 3 [78]. Brain tissue oxygen (PbtO2) and cerebral microdialysis can be used for individualized patient care vis-à-vis the above mechanisms of injury from local and regional hypoxia. Trend analysis of PbtO2 helps distinguish early from delayed injury, where a drop in PbtO2 has been shown to correlate with vasospasm and DCI [10]. Cerebral microdialysis can give data on the brain's metabolic profile that can be affected days before the irreversible injury [10]. The lactate-to-pyruvate ratio (LPR) has been studied as a potential biomarker in aSAH and other neurologic injuries. An increase in the LPR can be associated with ischemia and poor patient outcomes [79]. A recent study [80] used a multimodal approach to create a useful diagnostic tool to detect patients at risk for ischemia. A fraction of inspired oxygen (FiO2) challenge was completed that would normally increase the PbtO2. The investigators noted that patients with higher cerebral lactate had less increase in PbtO2 and concluded that a less-than-expected increase in PbtO2 vis-à-vis FiO2 challenge could be a surrogate for elevated cerebral lactate and risk for ischemia. Megjhani et al. [81] measured CPP in association with PbtO2. A non-linear relationship was found, but it showed that hypoperfusion and less than optimal values of CPP were associated with decreased PbtO2 and regional brain hypoxia. Because of a nonstandard approach related to these modalities, studies of invasive multimodal monitoring have produced mixed results. The ability to interpret results, recognize, and treat patients based on those results are user and training-dependent. However, these tools demonstrate the focus on microcellular milieu data, contrasted with the previous thought of management based on large vessel vasospasm alone.

Table 2. Multimodal Advanced Neuromonitoring.

Neurophysiological Parameters	Subtypes and Notes
Cerebral Autoregulation	• Relies on multiple modalities to maintain preferred CPP • Helpful to have an arterial line and advanced hemodynamic monitoring system
Cerebral Blood Flow	• Transcranial Doppler • Thermal Diffusion Flowmetry (Thermal Clearance Method) • CT or MR perfusion • Positron emission tomography—rarely used in practice
Cerebral Oxygenation	• PbtO2 • NIRS • Jugular venous oximetry
Intracranial Pressure	• External ventricular drain—benefit of draining CSF as well as monitoring ICP • Parenchymal probe • Subdural ICP monitor
Electroencephalography (EEG)	• Conventional scalp EEG—non-invasive technique, easy to remove and replace • Subdural or depth electrodes
Pupillometry	• Abnormal decreases in NPi may be an early sign of DCI
Cerebral Microdialysis	• Clinical utility unclear

Table 3. Pathophysiologic Types of Cerebral Shock (adapted from Brain Shock-Toward Pathophysiologic Phenotyping in Traumatic Brain Injury [78]). Brain tissue oxygen (PbtO2); lactate/pyruvate ratio (LPR); cerebral blood flow (CBF); cerebral perfusion pressure (CPP); intracranial pressure (ICP); cortical spreading depression (CSD). If a neuromonitoring result is not listed, it is either unchanged or unpredictable.

Pathophysiologic Type	Neuromonitoring Result	Underlying Pathophysiology and Management
Flow Dependent	↓: PbtO2, glucose, pyruvate ↑: lactate, LPR	Suboptimal CBF → optimize hemodynamic parameters and CPP
Flow Independent Oxygen Diffusion Limitation	↓: PbtO2 ↑: lactate, LPR	Intracellular/interstitial edema → appropriately manage cerebral edema

Table 3. Cont.

Pathophysiologic Type	Neuromonitoring Result	Underlying Pathophysiology and Management
Flow Independent Energy Production (Mitochondrial) Failure	↓: lactate, LPR, possibly pyruvate ↑: glucose	Management is unclear
Flow Independent Microvascular Shunting	↓: PbtO2 (from ↑CBF) ↑: glucose, lactate	Microvascular shunting → appropriately manage ICP
Low Extraction	↓: PbtO2, pyruvate ↑: lactate, LPR	Hypoxemic, anemic or high-affinity hypoxia → treat appropriate underlying cause to improve oxygenation
Hypermetabolic	↓: PbtO2, glucose, pyruvate ↑: lactate, LPR Similar profile to flow dependent	Increase in metabolic demand → Avoid hyperthermia, seizures, CSD; consider sedation if appropriate

Near-infrared spectroscopy (NIRS) is a non-invasive brain tissue oxygenation monitoring device, but its use is limited due to the ability to monitor mainly the frontal lobe. De Courson et al. looked at the correlation between PbtO2 and NIRS measurements among 51 SAH patients and found no correlation [82]. Pupillometry has been well studied as a tool for early detection of potential worsening in brain injury cases. Regarding aSAH, Aoun et al. [83] looked at 56 patients with transcranial doppler and Neurological Pupil index (NPi) measurements in combination. In this study, sonographic vasospasm was not significantly associated with the NPi measurement, but sonographic vasospasm and abnormal decreases in NPi were each associated with DCI.

Cortical spreading depolarization and depression can be monitored along with continuous electroencephalogram (cEEG) to detect changes such as decreasing relative alpha variability, decreasing alpha-delta ratio, worsening focal slowing, or late-appearing epileptiform abnormalities that are considered EEG alarms [84–86]. This approach [85,86] could predict DCI days before the actual event, which is an exciting advancement and also shows this as a dynamic pathophysiologic process.

Vasospasm does occur around the period of DCI and cerebral infarction, though not always found to correlate with location or degree of ischemia. Transcranial Doppler is a non-invasive tool that can detect possible vasospasm. Mean flow velocities in the middle and anterior cerebral arteries are typically considered abnormal for >120 cm/s, with >200 cm/s consistent with severe vasospasm [10]. CT angiogram is another valuable non-invasive imaging modality that can be used for diagnosing cerebral vasospasm. However, catheter-based angiography remains the gold standard, giving both the ability to diagnose and treat. CT perfusion (CTP) imaging has been studied as a potential tool in detecting DCI. In a systematic review that included 345 patients, aSAH patients with perfusion deficits on CTP imaging demonstrated an approximately 23-fold higher likelihood of developing DCI than patients with normal CTP results [87]. Further, a mean transit time (MTT) exceeding 6.4 s, or regional CBF below 25 mL/100 g/min correlated with the development of DCI in the study [88]. In another study by Cremers et al. [89], aSAH patients with assessed perfusion deficit with CTP at the time of clinical deterioration were more often noted to develop infarction on follow-up imaging (88%) as compared with patients without a perfusion deficit (38%). CTP imaging can provide detailed information on microvascular circulation. Therefore, its combination with CT angiography or digital subtraction angiography can provide a complete view of cerebral circulation [90–93]. However, due to high variability in post-processing methods and equipment used, along with inconsistency with quantitative variables and their thresholds for detecting DCI, the question of the sensitivity of CTP is a question of clinicians [94]. Further prospective studies are required before the wide acceptance of CTP as a promising tool in detecting DCI.

5. Future Directions

Clinical and Risk Factor Assessment

Several studies have resulted in different grading systems based on clinical or radiological factors to predict DCI or outcomes to guide treatment [95]. The GCS, HH, and WFNS are the widely used clinical grading scales, focusing on signs and symptoms; however, these grading structures do not take into account the quantity and severity of bleeding. With the improved CT techniques, some radiographic scales have been further developed. Quantifying thickness and area of subarachnoid blood on CT scans, the Fisher Scale and the modified Fisher Scale can predict the incidence of cerebral vasospasm and DCI [7]. The SEBES is a new scoring tool that displays the degree of EBI to predict the incidence of DCI. However, further research is needed to determine its accuracy and effectiveness [64]. The main issue with radiological scales is the absence of clinical symptoms. Thus, a few combined grading systems have been promoted, including VASOGRADE (VG) [96] and the HAIR [97] scales described in Table 4, to predict DCI and in-hospital mortality respectively [97]. However, those grading structures do not consider the importance of EBI. New studies have recognized that the incidence of DCI is associated with the severity of EBI after SAH [98]. Other scores include combining multiple variables of admission data [99] and more dynamic scores to give clinicians insight into the possibility of current DCI [100].

Table 4. VASOGRADE and HAIR scores, from respective studies, for aneurysmal subarachnoid hemorrhage. Modified Fisher scale (mF), World Federation of Neurosurgical Societies scale (WFNS); Hunt and Hess score (HH); Intraventricular hemorrhage (IVH).

Score	Purpose	Score components	Findings
VASOGRADE (N = 746)	DCI risk stratification	Green: mF 1–2 AND WFNS 1–2 Yellow: mF 3–4 AND WFNS 1–3 Red: WFNS 4–5 regardless of mF grade	Yellow: tendency to DCI compared to Green Red: 3-fold increased risk of DCI compared to Green
HAIR (N = 400–score development) (N = 302 –score validation)	In-hospital mortality risk stratification	Score 0–8 total HH: 1–3 = 0 pts; 4 = 1 pt; 5 = 4 pts Age: <60 = 0 pts; 60–80 = 1 pt; ≥80 = 2 pts IVH: No = 0 pts; Yes = 1 pt Re-bleed (within 24hrs): No = 0 pts; Yes = 1 pt	Increase in HAIR score increase in rate of in-hospital mortality

Multiple predictive models have been recommended for DCI. Coated platelets, a subset of platelet that keeps the prothrombotic substance attached to the platelet and a marker for thrombogenicity, was studied to look at DCI prediction. The trend of coated platelets after initial ictus was found to be a reliable predictor of DCI [101]. Machine-learning capabilities for better prediction have been shown to be beneficial in multiple studies and are promising roads for future research [102,103].

6. Necessity for Ongoing Research

Further reliable predictive models and markers to determine patients at high risk for DCI and other complications following aSAH are an important continued endeavor. As mentioned previously regarding genetic predisposition to DCI, the potential of polymorphisms associated with nitric oxide synthase (NOS), specifically the neuronal type, has shown promising bench research results. Endothelial NOS was not significantly shown to increase DCI or vasospasm risk in a meta-analysis [28]. Although challenging due to the unavailability of either pre- or post-morbid genetic testing, further prospective studies may shed a better light on the role of endothelial NOS.

The oxidative stress associated with the initial catecholamine surge at the ictus has been studied vis-à-vis possible mechanisms to address the complications arising from that excitatory response. Renal denervation was investigated to stabilize the sympathetic response by deactivating efferent sympathetic nerves in the periphery. This reduced angiotensin-II and endothelin-1 in animal models and offered hope for inhibiting vasoconstriction and vasospasm [45]. Although previous studies have proven that treatment of vasospasm may not improve outcomes, the idea of continued research to address the ictal sympathetic surge is possible.

A multicenter study with a large sample size and standardized variables is needed regarding aSAH to find the best generalizable and reproducible results to lead to a change in clinical practice. Using relevant preclinical models is an essential part of conducting translational studies [104]. This is necessary to address the limited treatment options that currently exist for aSAH and DCI with a significant degree of poor outcomes.

7. Conclusions

The primary goal of neurointensivists in clinical practice is to ameliorate the burden of morbidity and mortality associated with aSAH. DCI is a complex multifactorial pathophysiological process that starts early post-aSAH, with risk factors present before and at ictus. The pathophysiology of EBI and the mechanisms mentioned earlier act as a substrate for the development of DCI. This includes the well-known mechanism of vasoconstriction and spasm, focusing on the sympathetic surge and cytokine release, microthrombosis, and BBB breakdown. Early focus on EBI and global cerebral edema are essential in managing aSAH. Our research goals should continue to change and attempt to address these newer pathomechanisms in a search for improved outcomes that can be translated into routine clinical practice.

Funding: This research received no external funding.

Institutional Review Board Statement: Not applicable.

Informed Consent Statement: Not applicable.

Data Availability Statement: Data sharing not applicable.

Acknowledgments: Divani's studies are funded by the UNM Center for Brain Recovery and Repair Center of Biomedical Research Excellence through Grant Number NIH P20GM109089 (Pilot PI), W81XWH-17-2-0053 (PI), and 1R21NS130423-01 (PI).

Conflicts of Interest: The authors declare no conflict of interest.

Abbreviations

aSAH	Aneurysmal subarachnoid hemorrhage
ADC	Apparent diffusion coefficient
APOE	Apolipoprotein E
CBF	Cerebral blood flow
CPP	Cerebral perfusion pressure
CT	Computed tomography
DCI	Delayed cerebral ischemia
EBI	Early brain injury
EEG	Electroencephalogram
eNOS	Endothelial nitric oxide synthase
EWAS	Epigenome wide association studies
FiO2	Fraction of inspired oxygen
GCS	Glasgow Coma Scale
GWAS	genome wide association studies
Hp	Haptoglobin
ICP	Intracranial pressure
IL-6	Interleukin 6
MAP	Mean arterial pressure

MIF	Macrophage migratory inhibitory factor
MRI	Magnetic resonance imaging
NIHSS	National Institute of Health Stroke Scale
NIRS	Near-infrared spectroscopy
NOS	Nitric oxide synthase
Npi	Neurological Pupil index
NRG1	Neuregulin 1
OR	Odds ratio
PbtO2	Brain tissue oxygenation
PRS	Polygenic risk scores
RYY-1	Ryanodine-1
SEBES	Subarachnoid hemorrhage early brain edema score
wPRS	Weighted PRS

References

1. Etminan, N.; Chang, H.S.; Hackenberg, K.; de Rooij, N.K.; Vergouwen, M.D.I.; Rinkel, G.J.E.; Algra, A. Worldwide Incidence of Aneurysmal Subarachnoid Hemorrhage According to Region, Time Period, Blood Pressure, and Smoking Prevalence in the Population: A Systematic Review and Meta-analysis. *JAMA Neurol.* 2019, 76, 588–597. [CrossRef]
2. De Oliveira Manoel, A.L.; Mansur, A.; Silva, G.S.; Germans, M.R.; Jaja, B.N.; Kouzmina, E.; Marotta, T.R.; Abrahamson, S.; Schweizer, T.A.; Spears, J.; et al. Functional Outcome After Poor-Grade Subarachnoid Hemorrhage: A Single-Center Study and Systematic Literature Review. *Neurocritical Care* 2016, 25, 338–350. [CrossRef] [PubMed]
3. Nieuwkamp, D.J.; Setz, L.E.; Algra, A.; Linn, F.H.; de Rooij, N.K.; Rinkel, G.J. Changes in case fatality of aneurysmal subarachnoid haemorrhage over time, according to age, sex, and region: A meta-analysis. *Lancet Neurol.* 2009, 8, 635–642. [CrossRef]
4. Springer, M.V.; Schmidt, J.M.; Wartenberg, K.E.; Frontera, J.A.; Badjatia, N.; Mayer, S.A. Predictors of global cognitive impairment 1 year after subarachnoid hemorrhage. *Neurosurgery* 2009, 65, 1043–1050. [CrossRef]
5. Geraghty, J.R.; Testai, F.D. Delayed Cerebral Ischemia after Subarachnoid Hemorrhage: Beyond Vasospasm and Towards a Multifactorial Pathophysiology. *Curr. Atheroscler. Rep.* 2017, 19, 50. [CrossRef]
6. Adams, H.P., Jr.; Kassell, N.F.; Torner, J.C.; Haley, E.C., Jr. Predicting cerebral ischemia after aneurysmal subarachnoid hemorrhage: Influences of clinical condition, CT results, and antifibrinolytic therapy. A report of the Cooperative Aneurysm Study. *Neurology* 1987, 37, 1586–1591. [CrossRef]
7. Frontera, J.A.; Claassen, J.; Schmidt, J.M.; Wartenberg, K.E.; Temes, R.; Connolly, E.S., Jr.; MacDonald, R.L.; Mayer, S.A. Prediction of symptomatic vasospasm after subarachnoid hemorrhage: The modified fisher scale. *Neurosurgery* 2006, 59, 21–27. [CrossRef]
8. Francoeur, C.L.; Mayer, S.A. Management of delayed cerebral ischemia after subarachnoid hemorrhage. *Crit. Care* 2016, 20, 277. [CrossRef] [PubMed]
9. Saripalli, M.; Tan, D.; Chandra, R.V.; Lai, L.T. Predictive Relevance of Early Temperature Elevation on the Risk of Delayed Cerebral Ischemia Development Following Aneurysmal Subarachnoid Hemorrhage. *World Neurosurg.* 2021, 150, e474–e481. [CrossRef] [PubMed]
10. Rass, V.; Helbok, R. How to diagnose delayed cerebral ischaemia and symptomatic vasospasm and prevent cerebral infarction in patients with subarachnoid haemorrhage. *Curr. Opin. Crit. Care* 2021, 27, 103–114. [CrossRef]
11. Ikram, A.; Javaid, M.A.; Ortega-Gutierrez, S.; Selim, M.; Kelangi, S.; Anwar, S.M.H.; Torbey, M.T.; Divani, A.A. Delayed Cerebral Ischemia after Subarachnoid Hemorrhage. *J. Stroke Cerebrovasc. Dis.* 2021, 30, 106064. [CrossRef]
12. Schmidt, T.P.; Weiss, M.; Hoellig, A.; Nikoubashman, O.; Schulze-Steinen, H.; Albanna, W.; Clusmann, H.; Schubert, G.A.; Veldeman, M. Revisiting the Timeline of Delayed Cerebral Ischemia After Aneurysmal Subarachnoid Hemorrhage: Toward a Temporal Risk Profile. *Neurocritical Care* 2022, 37, 735–743. [CrossRef] [PubMed]
13. Rosengart, A.J.; Schultheiss, K.E.; Tolentino, J.; Macdonald, R.L. Prognostic factors for outcome in patients with aneurysmal subarachnoid hemorrhage. *Stroke J. Cereb. Circ.* 2007, 38, 2315–2321. [CrossRef]
14. Vergouwen, M.D.; Vermeulen, M.; van Gijn, J.; Rinkel, G.J.; Wijdicks, E.F.; Muizelaar, J.P.; Mendelow, A.D.; Juvela, S.; Yonas, H.; Terbrugge, K.G.; et al. Definition of delayed cerebral ischemia after aneurysmal subarachnoid hemorrhage as an outcome event in clinical trials and observational studies: Proposal of a multidisciplinary research group. *Stroke J. Cereb. Circ.* 2010, 41, 2391–2395. [CrossRef] [PubMed]
15. Raatikainen, E.; Vahtera, A.; Kuitunen, A.; Junttila, E.; Huhtala, H.; Ronkainen, A.; Pyysalo, L.; Kiiski, H. Prognostic value of the 2010 consensus definition of delayed cerebral ischemia after aneurysmal subarachnoid hemorrhage. *J. Neurol. Sci.* 2021, 420, 117261. [CrossRef]
16. Etminan, N.; Vergouwen, M.D.; Macdonald, R.L. Angiographic vasospasm versus cerebral infarction as outcome measures after aneurysmal subarachnoid hemorrhage. *Acta Neurochir. Suppl.* 2013, 115, 33–40. [CrossRef]
17. Foreman, B. The Pathophysiology of Delayed Cerebral Ischemia. *J. Clin. Neurophysiol.* 2016, 33, 174–182. [CrossRef] [PubMed]

18. Macdonald, R.L.; Higashida, R.T.; Keller, E.; Mayer, S.A.; Molyneux, A.; Raabe, A.; Vajkoczy, P.; Wanke, I.; Bach, D.; Frey, A.; et al. Clazosentan, an endothelin receptor antagonist, in patients with aneurysmal subarachnoid haemorrhage undergoing surgical clipping: A randomised, double-blind, placebo-controlled phase 3 trial (CONSCIOUS-2). *Lancet Neurol.* **2011**, *10*, 618–625. [CrossRef]
19. Ya, X.; Zhang, C.; Zhang, S.; Zhang, Q.; Cao, Y.; Wang, S.; Zhao, J. The Relationship Between Smoking and Delayed Cerebral Ischemia After Intracranial Aneurysm Rupture: A Systematic Review and Meta-Analysis. *Front. Neurol.* **2021**, *12*, 625087. [CrossRef]
20. Duan, W.; Pan, Y.; Wang, C.; Wang, Y.; Zhao, X.; Wang, Y.; Liu, L.; CNSR Investigators. Risk Factors and Clinical Impact of Delayed Cerebral Ischemia after Aneurysmal Subarachnoid Hemorrhage: Analysis from the China National Stroke Registry. *Neuroepidemiology* **2018**, *50*, 128–136. [CrossRef]
21. Crobeddu, E.; Mittal, M.K.; Dupont, S.; Wijdicks, E.F.; Lanzino, G.; Rabinstein, A.A. Predicting the lack of development of delayed cerebral ischemia after aneurysmal subarachnoid hemorrhage. *Stroke J. Cereb. Circ.* **2012**, *43*, 697–701. [CrossRef] [PubMed]
22. Bakker, M.K.; Ruigrok, Y.M. Genetics of Intracranial Aneurysms. *Stroke J. Cereb. Circ.* **2021**, *52*, 3004–3012. [CrossRef]
23. Gaastra, B.; Alexander, S.; Bakker, M.K.; Bhagat, H.; Bijlenga, P.; Blackburn, S.; Collins, M.K.; Dore, S.; Griessenauer, C.; Hendrix, P.; et al. Genome-Wide Association Study of Clinical Outcome After Aneurysmal Subarachnoid Haemorrhage: Protocol. *Transl. Stroke Res.* **2022**, *13*, 565–576. [CrossRef] [PubMed]
24. Rinkel, G.J. Intracranial aneurysm screening: Indications and advice for practice. *Lancet Neurol.* **2005**, *4*, 122–128. [CrossRef] [PubMed]
25. Korja, M.; Silventoinen, K.; McCarron, P.; Zdravkovic, S.; Skytthe, A.; Haapanen, A.; de Faire, U.; Pedersen, N.L.; Christensen, K.; Koskenvuo, M.; et al. Genetic epidemiology of spontaneous subarachnoid hemorrhage: Nordic Twin Study. *Stroke J. Cereb. Circ.* **2010**, *41*, 2458–2462. [CrossRef]
26. Bakker, M.K.; van der Spek, R.A.A.; van Rheenen, W.; Morel, S.; Bourcier, R.; Hostettler, I.C.; Alg, V.S.; van Eijk, K.R.; Koido, M.; Akiyama, M.; et al. Genome-wide association study of intracranial aneurysms identifies 17 risk loci and genetic overlap with clinical risk factors. *Nat. Genet.* **2020**, *52*, 1303–1313. [CrossRef]
27. Theodotou, C.B.; Snelling, B.M.; Sur, S.; Haussen, D.C.; Peterson, E.C.; Elhammady, M.S. Genetic associations of intracranial aneurysm formation and sub-arachnoid hemorrhage. *Asian J. Neurosurg.* **2017**, *12*, 374–381. [CrossRef]
28. Solodovnikova, Y.; Ivaniuk, A.; Marusich, T.; Son, A. Meta-analysis of associations of genetic polymorphisms with cerebral vasospasm and delayed cerebral ischemia after aneurysmal subarachnoid hemorrhage. *Acta Neurol. Belg.* **2021**, *122*, 1547–1556. [CrossRef]
29. Gaastra, B.; Ren, D.; Alexander, S.; Bennett, E.R.; Bielawski, D.M.; Blackburn, S.L.; Borsody, M.K.; Dore, S.; Galea, J.; Garland, P.; et al. Haptoglobin genotype and aneurysmal subarachnoid hemorrhage: Individual patient data analysis. *Neurology* **2019**, *92*, e2150–e2164. [CrossRef]
30. Gaastra, B.; Glazier, J.; Bulters, D.; Galea, I. Haptoglobin Genotype and Outcome after Subarachnoid Haemorrhage: New Insights from a Meta-Analysis. *Oxid. Med. Cell. Longev.* **2017**, *2017*, 6747940. [CrossRef]
31. McInnes, M.D.; Bossuyt, P.M. Pitfalls of Systematic Reviews and Meta-Analyses in Imaging Research. *Radiology* **2015**, *277*, 13–21. [CrossRef] [PubMed]
32. Baumann, A.; Devaux, Y.; Audibert, G.; Zhang, L.; Bracard, S.; Colnat-Coulbois, S.; Klein, O.; Zannad, F.; Charpentier, C.; Longrois, D.; et al. Gene expression profile of blood cells for the prediction of delayed cerebral ischemia after intracranial aneurysm rupture: A pilot study in humans. *Cerebrovasc. Dis.* **2013**, *36*, 236–242. [CrossRef]
33. Kim, B.J.; Kim, Y.; Youn, D.H.; Park, J.J.; Rhim, J.K.; Kim, H.C.; Kang, K.; Jeon, J.P. Genome-wide blood DNA methylation analysis in patients with delayed cerebral ischemia after subarachnoid hemorrhage. *Sci. Rep.* **2020**, *10*, 11419. [CrossRef] [PubMed]
34. Heinsberg, L.W.; Weeks, D.E.; Alexander, S.A.; Minster, R.L.; Sherwood, P.R.; Poloyac, S.M.; Deslouches, S.; Crago, E.A.; Conley, Y.P. Iron homeostasis pathway DNA methylation trajectories reveal a role for STEAP3 metalloreductase in patient outcomes after aneurysmal subarachnoid hemorrhage. *Epigenetics Commun.* **2021**, *1*, 4. [CrossRef]
35. Guttmacher, A.E.; Porteous, M.E.; McInerney, J.D. Educating health-care professionals about genetics and genomics. *Nat. Rev. Genet.* **2007**, *8*, 151–157. [CrossRef] [PubMed]
36. Torkamani, A.; Wineinger, N.E.; Topol, E.J. The personal and clinical utility of polygenic risk scores. *Nat. Rev. Genet.* **2018**, *19*, 581–590. [CrossRef]
37. Slunecka, J.L.; van der Zee, M.D.; Beck, J.J.; Johnson, B.N.; Finnicum, C.T.; Pool, R.; Hottenga, J.J.; de Geus, E.J.C.; Ehli, E.A. Implementation and implications for polygenic risk scores in healthcare. *Hum. Genom.* **2021**, *15*, 46. [CrossRef]
38. Hong, E.P.; Youn, D.H.; Kim, B.J.; Lee, J.J.; Na, D.; Ahn, J.H.; Park, J.J.; Rhim, J.K.; Kim, H.C.; Jeon, H.J.; et al. Genome-wide polygenic risk impact on intracranial aneurysms and acute ischemic stroke. *PLoS ONE* **2022**, *17*, e0265581. [CrossRef]
39. Sehba, F.A.; Pluta, R.M.; Macdonald, R.L. Brain injury after transient global cerebral ischemia and subarachnoid hemorrhage. *Stroke Res. Treat.* **2013**, *2013*, 827154. [CrossRef]
40. Weimer, J.M.; Jones, S.E.; Frontera, J.A. Acute Cytotoxic and Vasogenic Edema after Subarachnoid Hemorrhage: A Quantitative MRI Study. *AJNR Am. J. Neuroradiol.* **2017**, *38*, 928–934. [CrossRef]
41. Hasegawa, Y.; Uchikawa, H.; Kajiwara, S.; Morioka, M. Central sympathetic nerve activation in subarachnoid hemorrhage. *J. Neurochem.* **2022**, *160*, 34–50. [CrossRef]
42. Crompton, M.R. Hypothalamic lesions following the rupture of cerebral berry aneurysms. *Brain* **1963**, *86*, 301–314. [CrossRef]

43. Lee, S.J.; Jang, S.H. Hypothalamic injury in spontaneous subarachnoid hemorrhage: A diffusion tensor imaging study. *Clin. Auton. Res.* **2021**, *31*, 321–322. [CrossRef]
44. Naredi, S.; Lambert, G.; Eden, E.; Zall, S.; Runnerstam, M.; Rydenhag, B.; Friberg, P. Increased sympathetic nervous activity in patients with nontraumatic subarachnoid hemorrhage. *Stroke J. Cereb. Circ.* **2000**, *31*, 901–906. [CrossRef] [PubMed]
45. Takemoto, Y.; Hasegawa, Y.; Hayashi, K.; Cao, C.; Hamasaki, T.; Kawano, T.; Mukasa, A.; Kim-Mitsuyama, S. The Stabilization of Central Sympathetic Nerve Activation by Renal Denervation Prevents Cerebral Vasospasm after Subarachnoid Hemorrhage in Rats. *Transl. Stroke Res.* **2020**, *11*, 528–540. [CrossRef] [PubMed]
46. Kawakita, F.; Kanamaru, H.; Asada, R.; Suzuki, Y.; Nampei, M.; Nakajima, H.; Oinaka, H.; Suzuki, H. Roles of glutamate in brain injuries after subarachnoid hemorrhage. *Histol. Histopathol.* **2022**, *37*, 1041–1051. [CrossRef]
47. Wan, W.H.; Ang, B.T.; Wang, E. The Cushing Response: A case for a review of its role as a physiological reflex. *J. Clin. Neurosci.* **2008**, *15*, 223–228. [CrossRef]
48. Schmidt, E.A.; Czosnyka, Z.; Momjian, S.; Czosnyka, M.; Bech, R.A.; Pickard, J.D. Intracranial baroreflex yielding an early cushing response in human. *Acta Neurochir. Suppl.* **2005**, *95*, 253–256. [CrossRef]
49. Chen, S.; Li, Q.; Wu, H.; Krafft, P.R.; Wang, Z.; Zhang, J.H. The harmful effects of subarachnoid hemorrhage on extracerebral organs. *Biomed. Res. Int.* **2014**, *2014*, 858496. [CrossRef]
50. Meyfroidt, G.; Baguley, I.J.; Menon, D.K. Paroxysmal sympathetic hyperactivity: The storm after acute brain injury. *Lancet Neurol.* **2017**, *16*, 721–729. [CrossRef] [PubMed]
51. Osgood, M.L. Aneurysmal Subarachnoid Hemorrhage: Review of the Pathophysiology and Management Strategies. *Curr. Neurol. Neurosci. Rep.* **2021**, *21*, 50. [CrossRef] [PubMed]
52. Calandra, T.; Bucala, R. Macrophage Migration Inhibitory Factor (MIF): A Glucocorticoid Counter-Regulator within the Immune System. *Crit. Rev. Immunol.* **2017**, *37*, 359–370. [CrossRef]
53. Chen, Y.H.; Cheng, Z.Y.; Shao, L.H.; Shentu, H.S.; Fu, B. Macrophage migration inhibitory factor as a serum prognostic marker in patients with aneurysmal subarachnoid hemorrhage. *Clin. Chim. Acta* **2017**, *473*, 60–64. [CrossRef]
54. Koda, M.; Nishio, Y.; Hashimoto, M.; Kamada, T.; Koshizuka, S.; Yoshinaga, K.; Onodera, S.; Nishihira, J.; Moriya, H.; Yamazaki, M. Up-regulation of macrophage migration-inhibitory factor expression after compression-induced spinal cord injury in rats. *Acta Neuropathol.* **2004**, *108*, 31–36. [CrossRef]
55. Su, Y.; Wang, Y.; Zhou, Y.; Zhu, Z.; Zhang, Q.; Zhang, X.; Wang, W.; Gu, X.; Guo, A.; Wang, Y. Macrophage migration inhibitory factor activates inflammatory responses of astrocytes through interaction with CD74 receptor. *Oncotarget* **2017**, *8*, 2719–2730. [CrossRef]
56. Inacio, A.R.; Ruscher, K.; Leng, L.; Bucala, R.; Deierborg, T. Macrophage migration inhibitory factor promotes cell death and aggravates neurologic deficits after experimental stroke. *J. Cereb. Blood Flow Metab.* **2011**, *31*, 1093–1106. [CrossRef]
57. Li, Y.S.; Chen, W.; Liu, S.; Zhang, Y.Y.; Li, X.H. Serum macrophage migration inhibitory factor levels are associated with infarct volumes and long-term outcomes in patients with acute ischemic stroke. *Int. J. Neurosci.* **2017**, *127*, 539–546. [CrossRef] [PubMed]
58. Yang, D.B.; Yu, W.H.; Dong, X.Q.; Zhang, Z.Y.; Du, Q.; Zhu, Q.; Che, Z.H.; Wang, H.; Shen, Y.F.; Jiang, L. Serum macrophage migration inhibitory factor concentrations correlate with prognosis of traumatic brain injury. *Clin. Chim. Acta* **2017**, *469*, 99–104. [CrossRef]
59. Lin, Q.; Cai, J.Y.; Lu, C.; Sun, J.; Ba, H.J.; Chen, M.H.; Chen, X.D.; Dai, J.X.; Lin, J.H. Macrophage migration inhibitory factor levels in serum from patients with acute intracerebral hemorrhage: Potential contribution to prognosis. *Clin. Chim. Acta* **2017**, *472*, 58–63. [CrossRef] [PubMed]
60. Yang, X.; Peng, J.; Pang, J.; Wan, W.; Zhong, C.; Peng, T.; Bao, K.; Jiang, Y. The Association Between Serum Macrophage Migration Inhibitory Factor and Delayed Cerebral Ischemia After Aneurysmal Subarachnoid Hemorrhage. *Neurotox. Res.* **2020**, *37*, 397–405. [CrossRef]
61. Hayman, E.G.; Wessell, A.; Gerzanich, V.; Sheth, K.N.; Simard, J.M. Mechanisms of Global Cerebral Edema Formation in Aneurysmal Subarachnoid Hemorrhage. *Neurocritical Care* **2017**, *26*, 301–310. [CrossRef]
62. Dreier, J.P.; Lemale, C.L.; Kola, V.; Friedman, A.; Schoknecht, K. Spreading depolarization is not an epiphenomenon but the principal mechanism of the cytotoxic edema in various gray matter structures of the brain during stroke. *Neuropharmacology* **2018**, *134*, 189–207. [CrossRef] [PubMed]
63. Wartenberg, K.E.; Sheth, S.J.; Michael Schmidt, J.; Frontera, J.A.; Rincon, F.; Ostapkovich, N.; Fernandez, L.; Badjatia, N.; Sander Connolly, E.; Khandji, A.; et al. Acute ischemic injury on diffusion-weighted magnetic resonance imaging after poor grade subarachnoid hemorrhage. *Neurocritical Care* **2011**, *14*, 407–415. [CrossRef]
64. Ahn, S.H.; Savarraj, J.P.; Pervez, M.; Jones, W.; Park, J.; Jeon, S.B.; Kwon, S.U.; Chang, T.R.; Lee, K.; Kim, D.H.; et al. The Subarachnoid Hemorrhage Early Brain Edema Score Predicts Delayed Cerebral Ischemia and Clinical Outcomes. *Neurosurgery* **2018**, *83*, 137–145. [CrossRef]
65. Sehba, F.A.; Hou, J.; Pluta, R.M.; Zhang, J.H. The importance of early brain injury after subarachnoid hemorrhage. *Prog. Neurobiol.* **2012**, *97*, 14–37. [CrossRef] [PubMed]
66. Pluta, R.M.; Hansen-Schwartz, J.; Dreier, J.; Vajkoczy, P.; Macdonald, R.L.; Nishizawa, S.; Kasuya, H.; Wellman, G.; Keller, E.; Zauner, A.; et al. Cerebral vasospasm following subarachnoid hemorrhage: Time for a new world of thought. *Neurol. Res.* **2009**, *31*, 151–158. [CrossRef]

67. Frontera, J.A.; Provencio, J.J.; Sehba, F.A.; McIntyre, T.M.; Nowacki, A.S.; Gordon, E.; Weimer, J.M.; Aledort, L. The Role of Platelet Activation and Inflammation in Early Brain Injury Following Subarachnoid Hemorrhage. *Neurocritical Care* **2017**, *26*, 48–57. [CrossRef] [PubMed]
68. Dreier, J.P.; Winkler, M.K.L.; Major, S.; Horst, V.; Lublinsky, S.; Kola, V.; Lemale, C.L.; Kang, E.J.; Maslarova, A.; Salur, I.; et al. Spreading depolarizations in ischaemia after subarachnoid haemorrhage, a diagnostic phase III study. *Brain* **2022**, *145*, 1264–1284. [CrossRef]
69. Owen, B.; Vangala, A.; Fritch, C.; Alsarah, A.A.; Jones, T.; Davis, H.; Shuttleworth, C.W.; Carlson, A.P. Cerebral Autoregulation Correlation with Outcomes and Spreading Depolarization in Aneurysmal Subarachnoid Hemorrhage. *Stroke J. Cereb. Circ.* **2022**, *53*, 1975–1983. [CrossRef]
70. Carlson, A.P.; Abbas, M.; Alunday, R.L.; Qeadan, F.; Shuttleworth, C.W. Spreading depolarization in acute brain injury inhibited by ketamine: A prospective, randomized, multiple crossover trial. *J. Neurosurg.* **2018**, *130*, 1513–1519. [CrossRef]
71. Reinhart, K.M.; Humphrey, A.; Brennan, K.C.; Carlson, A.P.; Shuttleworth, C.W. Memantine Improves Recovery After Spreading Depolarization in Brain Slices and can be Considered for Future Clinical Trials. *Neurocritical Care* **2021**, *35*, 135–145. [CrossRef] [PubMed]
72. Barber, P.A.; Demchuk, A.M.; Zhang, J.; Buchan, A.M. Validity and reliability of a quantitative computed tomography score in predicting outcome of hyperacute stroke before thrombolytic therapy. ASPECTS Study Group. Alberta Stroke Programme Early CT Score. *Lancet* **2000**, *355*, 1670–1674. [CrossRef] [PubMed]
73. Said, M.; Gumus, M.; Herten, A.; Dinger, T.F.; Chihi, M.; Darkwah Oppong, M.; Deuschl, C.; Wrede, K.H.; Kleinschnitz, C.; Sure, U.; et al. Subarachnoid Hemorrhage Early Brain Edema Score (SEBES) as a radiographic marker of clinically relevant intracranial hypertension and unfavorable outcome after subarachnoid hemorrhage. *Eur. J. Neurol.* **2021**, *28*, 4051–4059. [CrossRef] [PubMed]
74. Rass, V.; Ianosi, B.A.; Wegmann, A.; Gaasch, M.; Schiefecker, A.J.; Kofler, M.; Lindner, A.; Addis, A.; Almashad, S.S.; Rhomberg, P.; et al. Delayed Resolution of Cerebral Edema Is Associated with Poor Outcome After Nontraumatic Subarachnoid Hemorrhage. *Stroke J. Cereb. Circ.* **2019**, *50*, 828–836. [CrossRef]
75. Yuan, J.Y.; Chen, Y.; Kumar, A.; Zlepper, Z.; Jayaraman, K.; Aung, W.Y.; Clarke, J.V.; Allen, M.; Athiraman, U.; Osbun, J.; et al. Automated Quantification of Reduced Sulcal Volume Identifies Early Brain Injury After Aneurysmal Subarachnoid Hemorrhage. *Stroke J. Cereb. Circ.* **2021**, *52*, 1380–1389. [CrossRef]
76. Veldeman, M.; Albanna, W.; Weiss, M.; Conzen, C.; Schmidt, T.P.; Schulze-Steinen, H.; Wiesmann, M.; Clusmann, H.; Schubert, G.A. Invasive neuromonitoring with an extended definition of delayed cerebral ischemia is associated with improved outcome after poor-grade subarachnoid hemorrhage. *J. Neurosurg.* **2020**, *134*, 1527–1534. [CrossRef]
77. Veldeman, M.; Albanna, W.; Weiss, M.; Park, S.; Hoellig, A.; Clusmann, H.; Helbok, R.; Temel, Y.; Alexander Schubert, G. Invasive Multimodal Neuromonitoring in Aneurysmal Subarachnoid Hemorrhage: A Systematic Review. *Stroke J. Cereb. Circ.* **2021**, *52*, 3624–3632. [CrossRef]
78. Lazaridis, C. Brain Shock-Toward Pathophysiologic Phenotyping in Traumatic Brain Injury. *Crit. Care Explor.* **2022**, *4*, e0724. [CrossRef]
79. Zahra, K.; Gopal, N.; Freeman, W.D.; Turnbull, M.T. Using Cerebral Metabolites to Guide Precision Medicine for Subarachnoid Hemorrhage: Lactate and Pyruvate. *Metabolites* **2019**, *9*, 245. [CrossRef]
80. Hosmann, A.; Schnackenburg, P.; Rauscher, S.; Hopf, A.; Bohl, I.; Engel, A.; Brugger, J.; Graf, A.; Plochl, W.; Reinprecht, A.; et al. Brain Tissue Oxygen Response as Indicator for Cerebral Lactate Levels in Aneurysmal Subarachnoid Hemorrhage Patients. *J. Neurosurg. Anesthesiol.* **2022**, *34*, 193–200. [CrossRef]
81. Megjhani, M.; Weiss, M.; Ford, J.; Terilli, K.; Kastenholz, N.; Nametz, D.; Kwon, S.B.; Velazquez, A.; Agarwal, S.; Roh, D.J.; et al. Optimal Cerebral Perfusion Pressure and Brain Tissue Oxygen in Aneurysmal Subarachnoid Hemorrhage. *Stroke J. Cereb. Circ.* **2023**, *54*, 189–197. [CrossRef]
82. De Courson, H.; Proust-Lima, C.; Tuaz, E.; Georges, D.; Verchere, E.; Biais, M. Relationship Between Brain Tissue Oxygen and Near-Infrared Spectroscopy in Patients with Nontraumatic Subarachnoid Hemorrhage. *Neurocritical Care* **2022**, *37*, 620–628. [CrossRef]
83. Aoun, S.G.; Stutzman, S.E.; Vo, P.N.; El Ahmadieh, T.Y.; Osman, M.; Neeley, O.; Plitt, A.; Caruso, J.P.; Aiyagari, V.; Atem, F.; et al. Detection of delayed cerebral ischemia using objective pupillometry in patients with aneurysmal subarachnoid hemorrhage. *J. Neurosurg.* **2019**, *132*, 27–32. [CrossRef]
84. Yu, Z.; Wen, D.; Zheng, J.; Guo, R.; Li, H.; You, C.; Ma, L. Predictive Accuracy of Alpha-Delta Ratio on Quantitative Electroencephalography for Delayed Cerebral Ischemia in Patients with Aneurysmal Subarachnoid Hemorrhage: Meta-Analysis. *World Neurosurg.* **2019**, *126*, e510–e516. [CrossRef]
85. Baang, H.Y.; Chen, H.Y.; Herman, A.L.; Gilmore, E.J.; Hirsch, L.J.; Sheth, K.N.; Petersen, N.H.; Zafar, S.F.; Rosenthal, E.S.; Westover, M.B.; et al. The Utility of Quantitative EEG in Detecting Delayed Cerebral Ischemia After Aneurysmal Subarachnoid Hemorrhage. *J. Clin. Neurophysiol.* **2022**, *39*, 207–215. [CrossRef]
86. Rosenthal, E.S.; Biswal, S.; Zafar, S.F.; O'Connor, K.L.; Bechek, S.; Shenoy, A.V.; Boyle, E.J.; Shafi, M.M.; Gilmore, E.J.; Foreman, B.P.; et al. Continuous electroencephalography predicts delayed cerebral ischemia after subarachnoid hemorrhage: A prospective study of diagnostic accuracy. *Ann. Neurol.* **2018**, *83*, 958–969. [CrossRef]

87. Cremers, C.H.; van der Schaaf, I.C.; Wensink, E.; Greving, J.P.; Rinkel, G.J.; Velthuis, B.K.; Vergouwen, M.D. CT perfusion and delayed cerebral ischemia in aneurysmal subarachnoid hemorrhage: A systematic review and meta-analysis. *J. Cereb. Blood Flow Metab.* **2014**, *34*, 200–207. [CrossRef]
88. Mir, D.I.; Gupta, A.; Dunning, A.; Puchi, L.; Robinson, C.L.; Epstein, H.A.; Sanelli, P.C. CT perfusion for detection of delayed cerebral ischemia in aneurysmal subarachnoid hemorrhage: A systematic review and meta-analysis. *AJNR Am. J. Neuroradiol.* **2014**, *35*, 866–871. [CrossRef]
89. Cremers, C.H.; Vos, P.C.; van der Schaaf, I.C.; Velthuis, B.K.; Vergouwen, M.D.; Rinkel, G.J.; Dankbaar, J.W. CT perfusion during delayed cerebral ischemia after subarachnoid hemorrhage: Distinction between reversible ischemia and ischemia progressing to infarction. *Neuroradiology* **2015**, *57*, 897–902. [CrossRef]
90. Greenberg, E.D.; Gobin, Y.P.; Riina, H.; Johnson, C.E.; Tsiouris, A.J.; Comunale, J.; Sanelli, P.C. Role of CT perfusion imaging in the diagnosis and treatment of vasospasm. *Imaging Med.* **2011**, *3*, 287–297. [CrossRef]
91. Taran, S.; Mandell, D.M.; McCredie, V.A. CT Perfusion for the Detection of Delayed Cerebral Ischemia in the Presence of Neurologic Confounders. *Neurocritical Care* **2020**, *33*, 317–322. [CrossRef]
92. Shi, D.; Jin, D.; Cai, W.; Zhu, Q.; Dou, X.; Fan, G.; Shen, J.; Xu, L. Serial low-dose quantitative CT perfusion for the evaluation of delayed cerebral ischaemia following aneurysmal subarachnoid haemorrhage. *Clin. Radiol.* **2020**, *75*, 131–139. [CrossRef] [PubMed]
93. Dong, L.; Zhou, Y.; Wang, M.; Yang, C.; Yuan, Q.; Fang, X. Whole-brain CT perfusion on admission predicts delayed cerebral ischemia following aneurysmal subarachnoid hemorrhage. *Eur. J. Radiol.* **2019**, *116*, 165–173. [CrossRef] [PubMed]
94. Allen, J.W.; Prater, A.; Kallas, O.; Abidi, S.A.; Howard, B.M.; Tong, F.; Agarwal, S.; Yaghi, S.; Dehkharghani, S. Diagnostic Performance of Computed Tomography Angiography and Computed Tomography Perfusion Tissue Time-to-Maximum in Vasospasm Following Aneurysmal Subarachnoid Hemorrhage. *J. Am. Heart. Assoc.* **2022**, *11*, e023828. [CrossRef] [PubMed]
95. Rajajee, V. Grading scales in subarachnoid hemorrhage—Many options, but do we have a winner? *Eur. J. Neurol.* **2018**, *25*, 207–208. [CrossRef]
96. De Oliveira Manoel, A.L.; Jaja, B.N.; Germans, M.R.; Yan, H.; Qian, W.; Kouzmina, E.; Marotta, T.R.; Turkel-Parrella, D.; Schweizer, T.A.; Macdonald, R.L.; et al. The VASOGRADE: A Simple Grading Scale for Prediction of Delayed Cerebral Ischemia After Subarachnoid Hemorrhage. *Stroke J. Cereb. Circ.* **2015**, *46*, 1826–1831. [CrossRef]
97. Lee, V.H.; Ouyang, B.; John, S.; Conners, J.J.; Garg, R.; Bleck, T.P.; Temes, R.E.; Cutting, S.; Prabhakaran, S. Risk stratification for the in-hospital mortality in subarachnoid hemorrhage: The HAIR score. *Neurocritical Care* **2014**, *21*, 14–19. [CrossRef]
98. Cahill, J.; Calvert, J.W.; Zhang, J.H. Mechanisms of early brain injury after subarachnoid hemorrhage. *J. Cereb. Blood Flow Metab.* **2006**, *26*, 1341–1353. [CrossRef]
99. Liu, H.; Xu, Q.; Li, A. Nomogram for predicting delayed cerebral ischemia after aneurysmal subarachnoid hemorrhage in the Chinese population. *J. Stroke Cerebrovasc. Dis.* **2020**, *29*, 105005. [CrossRef]
100. Megjhani, M.; Terilli, K.; Weiss, M.; Savarraj, J.; Chen, L.H.; Alkhachroum, A.; Roh, D.J.; Agarwal, S.; Connolly, E.S., Jr.; Velazquez, A.; et al. Dynamic Detection of Delayed Cerebral Ischemia: A Study in 3 Centers. *Stroke J. Cereb. Circ.* **2021**, *52*, 1370–1379. [CrossRef]
101. Ray, B.; Pandav, V.M.; Mathews, E.A.; Thompson, D.M.; Ford, L.; Yearout, L.K.; Bohnstedt, B.N.; Chaudhary, S.; Dale, G.L.; Prodan, C.I. Coated-Platelet Trends Predict Short-Term Clinical Outcome After Subarachnoid Hemorrhage. *Transl. Stroke Res.* **2018**, *9*, 459–470. [CrossRef]
102. Ramos, L.A.; van der Steen, W.E.; Sales Barros, R.; Majoie, C.; van den Berg, R.; Verbaan, D.; Vandertop, W.P.; Zijlstra, I.; Zwinderman, A.H.; Strijkers, G.J.; et al. Machine learning improves prediction of delayed cerebral ischemia in patients with subarachnoid hemorrhage. *J. Neurointerventional Surg.* **2019**, *11*, 497–502. [CrossRef]
103. Savarraj, J.P.J.; Hergenroeder, G.W.; Zhu, L.; Chang, T.; Park, S.; Megjhani, M.; Vahidy, F.S.; Zhao, Z.; Kitagawa, R.S.; Choi, H.A. Machine Learning to Predict Delayed Cerebral Ischemia and Outcomes in Subarachnoid Hemorrhage. *Neurology* **2021**, *96*, e553–e562. [CrossRef]
104. Goursaud, S.; de Lizarrondo, S.M.; Grolleau, F.; Chagnot, A.; Agin, V.; Maubert, E.; Gauberti, M.; Vivien, D.; Ali, C.; Gakuba, C. Delayed Cerebral Ischemia After Subarachnoid Hemorrhage: Is There a Relevant Experimental Model? A Systematic Review of Preclinical Literature. *Front. Cardiovasc. Med.* **2021**, *8*, 752769. [CrossRef]

Disclaimer/Publisher's Note: The statements, opinions and data contained in all publications are solely those of the individual author(s) and contributor(s) and not of MDPI and/or the editor(s). MDPI and/or the editor(s) disclaim responsibility for any injury to people or property resulting from any ideas, methods, instructions or products referred to in the content.

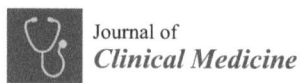

Journal of
Clinical Medicine

Article

Aneurysmal Subarachnoid Hemorrhage in Hospitalized Patients on Anticoagulants—A Two Center Matched Case-Control Study

Michael Veldeman [1,2,*], Tobias Rossmann [1,3], Miriam Weiss [2,4], Catharina Conzen-Dilger [2], Miikka Korja [1], Anke Hoellig [2], Jyri J. Virta [1,5], Jarno Satopää [1], Teemu Luostarinen [6], Hans Clusmann [2], Mika Niemelä [1] and Rahul Raj [1]

[1] Department of Neurosurgery, University of Helsinki and Helsinki University Hospital, 00260 Helsinki, Finland
[2] Department of Neurosurgery, RWTH Aachen University Hospital, 52074 Aachen, Germany
[3] Department of Neurosurgery, Neuromed Campus, Kepler University Hospital, 4021 Linz, Austria
[4] Department of Neurosurgery, Kantonsspital Aarau, 5001 Aarau, Switzerland
[5] Division of Anesthesiology, Department of Anesthesiology, Intensive Care and Pain Medicine, University of Helsinki and Helsinki University Hospital, 00260 Helsinki, Finland
[6] Anaesthesiology and Intensive Care, University of Helsinki and Helsinki University Hospital, 00260 Helsinki, Finland
* Correspondence: mveldeman@ukaachen.de; Tel.: +358-09-471-87409

Citation: Veldeman, M.; Rossmann, T.; Weiss, M.; Conzen-Dilger, C.; Korja, M.; Hoellig, A.; Virta, J.J.; Satopää, J.; Luostarinen, T.; Clusmann, H.; et al. Aneurysmal Subarachnoid Hemorrhage in Hospitalized Patients on Anticoagulants—A Two Center Matched Case-Control Study. *J. Clin. Med.* **2023**, *12*, 1476. https://doi.org/10.3390/jcm12041476

Academic Editor: Ramazan Jabbarli

Received: 6 January 2023
Revised: 30 January 2023
Accepted: 9 February 2023
Published: 13 February 2023

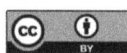

Copyright: © 2023 by the authors. Licensee MDPI, Basel, Switzerland. This article is an open access article distributed under the terms and conditions of the Creative Commons Attribution (CC BY) license (https:// creativecommons.org/licenses/by/ 4.0/).

Abstract: Objective—Direct oral anticoagulants (DOAC) are replacing vitamin K antagonists (VKA) for the prevention of ischemic stroke and venous thromboembolism. We set out to assess the effect of prior treatment with DOAC and VKA in patients with aneurysmal subarachnoid hemorrhage (SAH). **Methods**—Consecutive SAH patients treated at two (Aachen, Germany and Helsinki, Finland) university hospitals were considered for inclusion. To assess the association between anticoagulant treatments on SAH severity measure by modified Fisher grading (mFisher) and outcome as measured by the Glasgow outcome scale (GOS, 6 months), DOAC- and VKA-treated patients were compared against age- and sex-matched SAH controls without anticoagulants. **Results**—During the inclusion timeframes, 964 SAH patients were treated in both centers. At the time point of aneurysm rupture, nine patients (0.93%) were on DOAC treatment, and 15 (1.6%) patients were on VKA. These were matched to 34 and 55 SAH age- and sex-matched controls, re-spectively. Overall, 55.6% of DOAC-treated patients suffered poor-grade (WFNS$_{4-5}$) SAH compared to 38.2% among their respective controls ($p = 0.35$); 53.3% of patients on VKA suffered poor-grade SAH compared to 36.4% in their respective controls ($p = 0.23$). Neither treatment with DOAC (aOR 2.70, 95%CI 0.30 to 24.23; $p = 0.38$), nor VKA (aOR 2.78, 95%CI 0.63 to 12.23; $p = 0.18$) were inde-pendently associated with unfavorable outcome (GOS$_{1-3}$) after 12 months. **Conclusions**—Iatrogenic coagulopathy caused by DOAC or VKA was not associated with more severe radiological or clinical subarachnoid hemorrhage or worse clinical outcome in hospitalized SAH patients.

Keywords: subarachnoid hemorrhage; intracranial aneurysm; direct oral anticoagulants; vitamin K antagonists

1. Introduction

Direct oral anticoagulants (DOAC) are progressively replacing vitamin K antagonists (VKA) for the prevention of ischemic stroke and venous thromboembolism [1–4]. Their use eliminates the need for constant monitoring of coagulation status due to more predictable pharmacokinetics and fewer drug interactions compared to VKA [5].

In contrast to VKA's indirect anticoagulant effect, DOAC directly inhibits a single clotting enzyme, factor-Xa, in case of apixaban, edoxaban and rivaroxaban, and thrombin in case of dabigatran [6]. Their relatively short half-life (around 12 h) allows spontaneous reversal of effects when elective or subacute surgery is warranted [7,8]. Idarucizumab, a costly monoclonal antibody fragment, reverses the anticoagulant effects of dabigatran only [9]. Andexanet alfa was approved as a reversal agent for rivaroxaban and apixaban in 2018, and other candidate antidotes currently undergoing clinical testing will follow [10,11].

Patients carrying an intracranial aneurysm are at risk of aneurysm rupture causing subarachnoid hemorrhage (SAH) [12]. Depending on the morphology and orientation of the aneurysm, bleeding can extend into brain parenchyma or ventricular system, causing ICH or intraventricular hemorrhage (IVH). The resulting acute increase of intracranial pressure (ICP) induces a drop in cerebral perfusion and can cause transient intracranial circulatory arrest [13] or sudden death [14]. Bleeding ceases once a clot effectively plugs the rupture site, a process requiring platelet adherences alongside functioning coagulation for thrombus stabilization [15]. Survivors need occlusion of the offending aneurysm from its parent vessel either by endovascular or surgical means, to prevent rebleeding [16]. The risk of re-rupture is the highest within the first hours [17]. Waiting to treat until effects are reversed by drug metabolization, is not desirable in SAH patients.

In two case-control analyses, VKA was associated with an increased risk of SAH [18,19]. The effects of DOAC intake in comparison with VKA on the severity, course, and outcome of SAH have not been investigated. Iatrogenic coagulopathy is suspected to worsen clinical and radiological severity of bleeding and increase the risk profile of aneurysm occlusion procedures as well as treatment of associated acute hydrocephalus. We set out to assess the bleeding severity and outcome after SAH, in patients on VKA and DOAC, in a two-center observational cohort study.

2. Methods

2.1. Patient Population and Study Design

All consecutive SAH patients who were treated at two university hospitals between 2010 and 2019 (RWTH Aachen University Hospital, Aachen, Germany) and between 2014 and 2019 (Helsinki University Hospital, Helsinki, Finland) were considered for inclusion. Patients aged 18 years or older with confirmation of ruptured aneurysm in either CT- or conventional cerebral angiography were included. From 2014 onward, the prospective data collection in Aachen was part of a previously registered observational study (NCT02142166) and was approved by the local ethics committee of the Medical Faculty of RWTH Aachen University (EK 062/14). The Helsinki database was retrospectively collected (HUS/125/2018). Due to the retrospective data collection of the remainder of data, the need for patient consent was waived by both local institutional research committees. Relevant patient baseline and SAH-specific data were extracted from existing electronic health records. The intake of antithrombotic drugs at time of SAH, in form of either antiplatelet drugs, VKA or DOAC, was noted. Coagulation status on admission consisting of platelet count and prothrombin time (PT) expressed as International Normalized Ratio (INR) was extracted. Clinical state on admission was assigned as best GCS performance in 24 h and graded by means of the World Federation of Neurological Surgeons (WFNS) grading scale. Clinical severity was dichotomized into good-grade (WFNS$_{1-3}$) and poor-grade (WFNS$_{4-5}$) SAH.

2.2. Standard of Care

In both inclusion centers, occlusion of the offending aneurysm was aimed for within 48 h via either surgical clipping or endovascular occlusion (coiling, flow-diverter stenting, or WEB-device placement). All patients were observed in a dedicated neurointensive care unit. Anticoagulant effects of VKA were acutely reversed by application of a body weight-adjusted dose of PCC until reaching a minimum INR of 1.2 [20]. Before antidotes were available, DOAC-treated patients also received PCC, but since 2014, the effect of dabigatran was reversed with idarucizumab [21,22]. In case of acute hydrocephalus, an external ventricular drain was placed prior to aneurysm occlusion but after anticoagulant reversal. After aneurysm occlusion, all patients received a wake-up test after which neurological assessability was continuously strived for. All patients were prophylactically treated with oral or intravenous nimodipine. More elaborate institutional treatment algorithms have been published previously [23,24].

2.3. Design and Outcome Parameters

To assess the effect of prior DOAC treatment on SAH severity and outcome, DOAC-treated patients were age- and sex-matched to non-DOAC controls with the aim of correcting for confounding comorbidities associated with anticoagulant use. Patients using VKA or DOAC and patients not using any antithrombotics were matched based on age and sex.

The same procedure was repeated for patients on VKA. Controls were only selected from patients from the same institution which were neither on VKA/DOAC nor any other antithrombotic treatment. Primary outcome was defined as radiological hemorrhage severity as measured by the modified Fisher scale [25] with additional assessment of the presence of ICH. Secondary outcome was defined as clinical hemorrhage severity (WFNS) [26] in form of incidence of poor-grade (WFNS$_{4-5}$) SAH, occurrence of delayed cerebral ischemia (DCI), in-hospital mortality, and clinical outcome after 12 months as measured via the Glasgow outcome scale (GOS) [27]. The GOS was dichotomized into favorable (GOS$_{4-5}$) and unfavorable outcome (GOS$_{1-3}$). The standing definition of clinical DCI by Vergouwen et al. [28] was applied whenever possible, but for the unconscious patient, diagnosis was based on perfusion CT-imaging or multimodal neuromonitoring [23,24,29].

2.4. Statistical Analysis

Numerical data are presented as median and interquartile ranges (Q$_1$–Q$_3$) due to small subgroup sizes. Categorical variables are provided as absolute case numbers and percentages. For nominal data, either the χ^2-Test or Fisher's exact test was used as appropriate based on group size. For continuous data, the Mann–Whitney U Test was used. A 3–4:1 age- and sex-matching of cases to controls was performed using the "ccmatch" function in STATA 17 (StataCorp LCC, College Station, TX, USA) selecting controls for each case only from patients coming from the same institution of treatment. Factors associated with occurrence of unfavorable outcome were assessed in a logistic regression model. Explanatory variables were included based on univariate results presenting with p-value < 0.10 or based on clinical relevance. Variables were tested for outliers via plotting and multicollinearity was evaluated via the assessment of the Variance Inflation Factor with a cut-off of 2.5. Multivariable-adjusted odds ratios (aORs) for SAH were estimated by conditional logistic regression. The latter statistical analyses were performed using IBM SPSS Statistics 25 (IBM Inc., Chicago, IL, USA). Statistical significance was defined as a two-sided $p < 0.05$.

3. Results

3.1. Patient Inclusion and Baseline Characteristics

During the inclusion timeframes, 964 SAH patient were treated, of whom 595 were in Helsinki and 369 were in Aachen. Sixty-six patients with an initial moribund presentation, none of which was treated with anticoagulants, were excluded. Moribund presentation was defined as clinical brainstem herniation based on bilateral fixed pupils or global supratentorial ischemic injury on imaging. A total of nine patients (0.93%) received DOAC treatment before suffering SAH, of whom two patients were treated with apixaban, a single patient with dabigatran, and six patients with rivaroxaban. No patients on edoxaban were identified. Seven patients received DOAC for non-valvular atrial fibrillation and two patients due to a history of deep vein thrombosis. No patients in the DOAC-control group suffered from type 2 diabetes.

A total of 15 (1.6%) SAH patients on VKA at the time point of aneurysm rupture were identified. Thereof, three patients were on phenprocoumon and 12 patients were on warfarin, prescribed for atrial fibrillation in 13 patients, and in three patients for a history of pulmonary embolism. No patients anticoagulated for mechanical heart valves were identified. As expected, patients on VKA presented with higher initial INR (2.2 (1.4–3.0) vs. 1.1 (1.0–1.1); $p < 0.001$). From the remainder of patients, 34 age- and sex-matched controls for DOAC cases and 55 controls for VKA cases were identified. An inclusion flow-chart is presented as Figure 1.

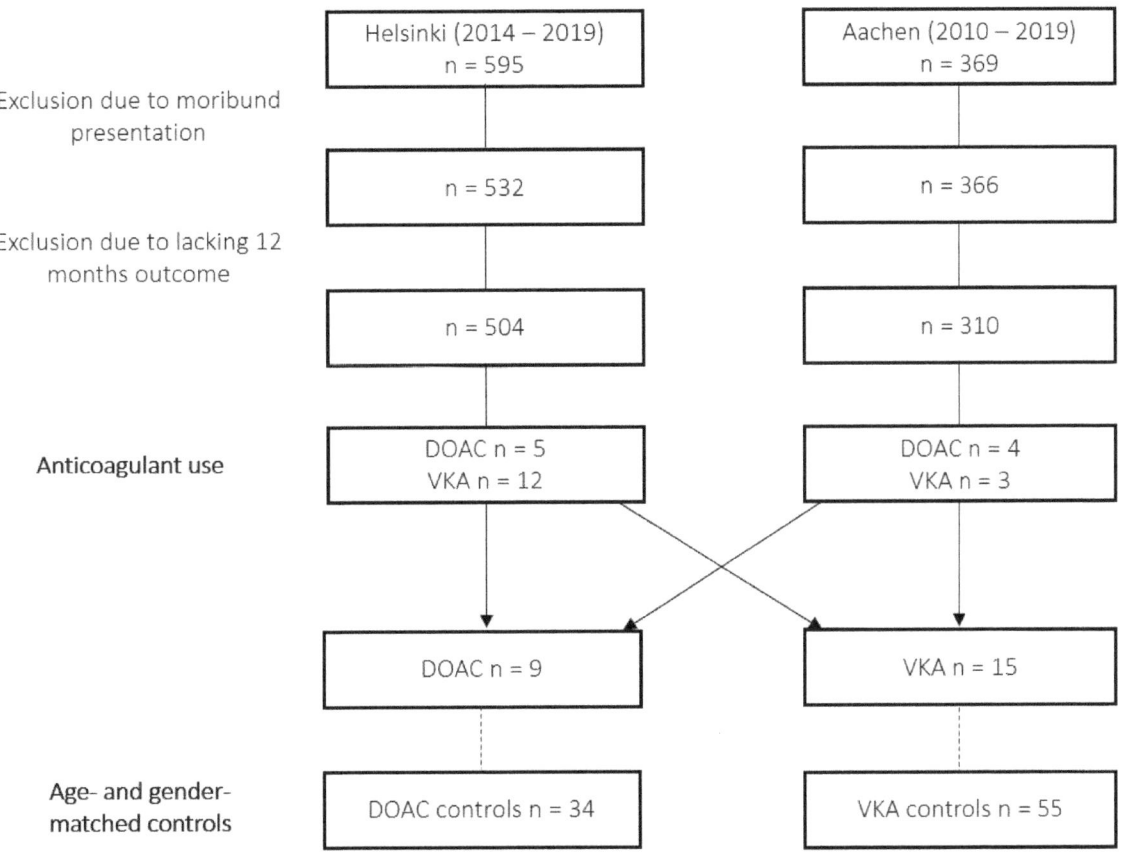

Figure 1. Inclusion flow-chart. DOAC, direct oral anticoagulant; VKA, vitamin K antagonist.

The location of the offending aneurysm was similarly distributed between both groups. Aneurysm distribution and size were comparable between VKA cases and controls. A comparison of patient baseline and SAH characteristics is presented in Tables 1 and 2.

3.2. Hemorrhage Severity

Radiological severity (modified Fisher scale) of SAH in patients on oral anticoagulants was similar compared to age- and sex-matched controls. Rates of IVH or ICH were not affected by intake of either DOAC or VKA (see Tables 1 and 2). A total of 55.6% of DOAC-treated patients suffered poor-grade SAH compared to 38.2% in the control group ($p = 0.349$). In SAH patients on VKA, 53.3% suffered poor-grade SAH vs. 36.4% in age- and sex-matched controls ($p = 0.234$). No patients with aneurysm rebleeding were identified.

Table 1. Comparison of patients on direct oral anticoagulants (DOAC) with age- and sex-matched controls without antithrombotic treatment.

	All (n = 43)	DOAC (n = 9)	Controls (n = 34)	*p*-Value
Demographics				
Age—yrs.—median (Q_1–Q_3)	67.5 (62.1–76.5)	66.6 (61.5–78.7)	68.1 (61.9–75.6)	0.895
Sex—Female/Male- no. (%)	25 (58.1)/18 (41.9)	5 (55.6)/4 (44.4)	20 (58.8)/14 (41.2)	0.860
Comorbidity—no. (%)				
Hypertension	26 (60.5)	5 (55.6)	21 (61.8)	0.735
Smoking	13 (30.2)	2 (22.2)	11 (32.4)	0.556
Diabetes type 2	2 (4.7)	2 (22.2)	0	n/a
Coronary artery disease	2 (4.7)	1 (11.1)	1 (2.9)	0.301
Coagulation status on admission				
INR—median (Q_1–Q_3)	1.1 (1.0–1.1)	1.1 (1.1–1.2)	1.0 (1.0–1.1)	0.081
Thrombocyte count (10^3/µL)—median (Q_1–Q_3)	241.0 (209.0–291.0)	235.0 (185.0–452.0)	243.5 (211.5–283.5)	0.895
Aneurysm location—no. (%)				
Acomm	16 (37.2)	4 (44.4)	12 (35.3)	0.256
MCA	10 (23.3)	1 (11.1)	9 (26.5)	
ICA (incl. Pcomm)	11 (25.6)	4 (44.4)	7 (20.6)	
Others	6 (14.0)	0 (0)	6 (17.6)	
Ant. circulation	37 (86.0)	9 (100.0)	28 (82.4)	0.174
Max. diameter (mm)—median (Q_1–Q_3)	6.0 (4.3–9.0)	5.0 (3.0–7.0)	7.0 (4.9–9.5)	0.135
Aneurysm occlusion—no. (%)				
Clipping/Endovascular	13 (30.2)/30 (69.8)	1 (11.1)/8 (88.9)	12 (35.3)/22 (64.7)	0.160
Hemorrhage severity				
WFNS grade—no. (%)				0.777
Grade 1	9 (20.9)	1 (11.1)	8 (23.5)	
Grade 2	10 (23.3)	2 (22.2)	8 (23.5)	
Grade 3	6 (14.0)	1 (11.1)	5 (14.7)	
Grade 4	6 (14.0)	1 (11.1)	5 (14.7)	
Grade 5	12 (27.9)	4 (44.4)	8 (23.5)	
Poor-grade SAH (WFNS$_{4-5}$)	18 (41.9)	5 (55.6)	13 (38.2)	0.349
Modified Fisher scale—no. (%)				0.558
Grade 1	8 (18.6)	1 (11.1)	7 (20.6)	
Grade 2	5 (11.6)	2 (22.2)	3 (8.8)	
Grade 3	9 (20.9)	1 (11.1)	8 (23.5)	
Grade 4	21 (48.8)	5 (55.6)	16 (47.1)	
IVH	26 (60.5)	7 (77.8)	19 (55.9)	0.296
ICH	15 (34.9)	4 (44.4)	11 (32.4)	0.499
Acute hydrocephalus	27 (62.8)	8 (88.9)	19 (55.9)	0.069

Acomm, aneurysm of the anterior communicating artery; ICH, intracerebral hemorrhage; INR, international normalized ratio; IVH, intraventricular hemorrhage; MCA, aneurysm of the middle cerebral artery; Pcomm, aneurysm of the posterior communicating artery; Q_1, first quartile; Q_3, third quartile; WFNS, World Federation of Neurological Surgeons.

3.3. Effects on Clinical Outcome

All patients on DOAC required mechanical ventilation (not including anesthesia for aneurysm occlusion) during their hospital stay compared to only 19 (55.9%) patients of matched controls ($p = 0.014$). The rate of patients suffering from sepsis, according to standing criteria, diagnosed by the presence of infection together with systemic manifestations of infection [30], was higher in patients who had received DOAC-treatment (n = 2 (22.2%) vs. n = 1 (2.9%); $p = 0.043$). No differences in the need for mechanical ventilation or the development of sepsis were noted between patients previously on VKA and matched controls. Six patients (66.7%) in the DOAC group compared to 19 (55.9%) controls were classified as unfavorable outcome after 12 months ($p = 0.560$). In VKA-treated patients,

11 (73.3%) patients were classified as unfavorable outcome compared to 26 (47.3%) patients in the matched control group (p = 0.073). An overview of clinical outcome parameters is presented in Table 3. Based on univariate logistic regression result (Supplementary Table S1), the association between previous DOAC treatment and unfavorable outcome (GOS$_{1-3}$) after 12 months was adjusted for WFNS grading, DCI occurrence, need for mechanical ventilation, and occurrence of sepsis. Introducing these explanatory variables into a conditional multivariable regression resulted in a significant model ($\chi^2(5)$ = 13.837, p = 0.017) explaining 36.7% (Nagelkerke R^2) of the variance in occurrence of unfavorable outcome and correctly classifying 74.4% of cases. Prior DOAC use was not independently associated with unfavorable outcome (aOR 2.696, 95%CI 0.300 to 24.228; p = 0.376).

Table 2. Comparison of patients on vitamin K antagonists (VKA) with age- and sex-matched controls without antithrombotic treatment.

	All (n = 70)	VKA (n = 15)	Controls (n = 55)	p-Value
Demographics				
Age—yrs.—median (Q_1–Q_3)	73.0 (65.0–76.8)	73.0 (66.4–76.6)	73.0 (63.8 - 77.6)	0.869
Sex—Female/Male- no. (%)	38 (54.3)/32 (45.7)	8 (53.3)/7 (46.7)	30 (54.5)/25 (45.5)	0.933
Comorbidity—no. (%)				
Hypertension	39 (55.7)	13 (86.7)	26 (47.3)	0.006
Smoking	17 (24.3)	3 (20.0)	14 (25.5)	0.662
Diabetes type 2	6 (8.6)	3 (20.0)	3 (5.5)	0.074
Coronary artery disease	3 (4.3)	3 (20.0)	0 (0)	**0.001**
Coagulation status on admission				
INR—median (Q_1–Q_3)	1.1 (1.0–1.2)	2.2 (1.4–3.0)	1.1 (1.0–1.1)	**<0.001**
Thrombocyte count (10^3/μL)—median (Q_1–Q_3)	241.0 (194.5–278.0)	221.0 (171.0–260.0)	242.0 (208.3–290.5)	0.169
Aneurysm location—no. (%)				
Acomm	23 (32.9)	5 (33.3)	18 (32.7)	0.094
MCA	16 (22.9)	2 (13.3)	14 (25.5)	
ICA (incl. Pcomm)	14 (20.0)	1 (6.7)	13 (23.6)	
Others	17 (24.3)	7 (46.7)	10 (18.2)	
Ant. circulation	53 (75.7)	8 (53.3)	45 (81.8)	0.023
Max. diameter (mm)—median (Q_1–Q_3)	6.0 (4.0–8.0)	6.2 (4.5–9.0)	6.0 (4.0–8.0)	0.873
Aneurysm occlusion—no. (%)				
Clipping/Endovascular	23 (32.9)/47 (67.1)	3 (20.0)/12 (80.0)	20 (36.4)/35 (63.6)	0.232
Hemorrhage severity				
WFNS grade—no. (%)				0.331
Grade 1	23 (32.9)	6 (40.0)	17 (30.9)	
Grade 2	9 (12.9)	1 (6.7)	8 (14.5)	
Grade 3	10 (14.3)	0 (0)	10 (18.2)	
Grade 4	12 (17.1)	3 (20.0)	9 (16.4)	
Grade 5	16 (22.9)	5 (33.3)	11 (20.0)	
Poor-grade SAH (WFNS$_{4-5}$)	28 (40.0)	8 (53.3)	20 (36.4)	0.234
Modified Fisher scale—no. (%)				0.528
Grade 1	11 (15.7)	2 (13.3)	9 (16.4)	
Grade 2	5 (7.1)	2 (13.3)	3 (5.5)	
Grade 3	17 (24.3)	2 (13.3)	15 (23.3)	
Grade 4	37 (52.9)	9 (60.0)	28 (50.9)	
IVH	40 (57.1)	11 (73.3)	29 (52.7)	0.153
ICH	22 (31.4)	5 (33.3)	17 (30.9)	0.858
Acute hydrocephalus	46 (65.7)	12 (80.0)	34 (61.8)	0.189

Acomm, aneurysm of the anterior communicating artery; ICH, intracerebral hemorrhage; INR, international normalized ratio; IVH, intraventricular hemorrhage; MCA, aneurysm of the middle cerebral artery; Pcomm, aneurysm of the posterior communicating artery; Q_1, first quartile; Q_3, third quartile; WFNS, World Federation of Neurological Surgeons. Significant p-values (<0.05) are marked in bold.

Table 3. Outcome comparison of patients on either direct oral anticoagulants (DOAC) or vitamin K antagonists (VKA) with age- and sex-matched controls without antithrombotic treatment.

	All (n = 43)	DOAC (n = 9)	Controls (n = 34)	*p*-Value
ICU-related complications				
Mechanical ventilation—no. (%)	28 (65.1)	9 (100)	19 (55.9)	0.014
Sepsis—no. (%)	3 (7.0)	2 (22.2)	1 (2.9)	0.043
DCI occurrence—no. (%)	15 (34.9%)	2 (22.2)	13 (38.2)	0.370
Clinical outcome				
In-hospital mortality—no. (%)	7 (16.3)	3 (33.3)	4 (11.8)	0.119
GOS 12 months—no. (%)				0.892
Good recovery	10 (23.3)	2 (22.2)	8 (23.5)	
Moderate disability	8 (18.6)	1 (11.1)	7 (20.6)	
Severe disability	14 (32.6)	3 (33.3)	11 (32.4)	
Vegetative state	1 (2.3)	0 (0)	1 (2.9)	
Dead	10 (23.3)	3 (33.3)	7 (20.6)	
Unfavorable outcome (GOS$_{1-3}$)	25 (58.1)	6 (66.7)	19 (55.9)	0.560
	All (n = 70)	VKA (n = 15)	Controls (n = 55)	*p*-Value
ICU-related complications				
Mechanical ventilation—no. (%)	50 (71.4)	38 (69.1)	12 (80.0)	0.407
Sepsis—no. (%)	9 (12.9)	7 (12.7)	2 (13.3)	0.950
DCI occurrence—no. (%)	21 (30.0)	17 (30.9)	4 (26.7)	0.751
Clinical outcome				
In hospital mortality—no. (%)	19 (27.1)	3 (20.0)	16 (29.1)	0.483
GOS 12 months—no. (%)				0.907
Good recovery	22 (31.4)	3 (20.0)	19 (34.5)	
Moderate disability	11 (15.7)	1 (6.7)	10 (18.2)	
Severe disability	13 (18.6)	6 (40.0)	7 (12.7)	
Vegetative state	3 (4.3)	1 (6.7)	2 (3.6)	
Dead	21 (30.0)	4 (26.7)	17 (30.9)	
Unfavorable outcome (GOS$_{1-3}$)	37 (52.9)	11 (73.3)	26 (47.3)	0.073

DCI, delayed cerebral ischemia; DOAC, direct oral anticoagulants; GOS, Glasgow outcome scale; ICU, intensive care unit; VKA, vitamin K antagonists.

A second model was built to assess the association between VKA use and unfavorable outcome resulting in a significant model ($\chi^2(5) = 26.364$, $p < 0.001$; Nagelkerke $R^2 = 0.419$) classifying 87.8% of cases correctly. Treatment with VKA had no effect on the occurrence of unfavorable outcome after 12 months (aOR 2.780, 95%CI 0.631 to 12.234; $p = 0.176$) (See Supplementary Table S2). Comparing the proportions of unfavorable outcome between DOAC and VKA patients yielded a $\chi^2(2)$ statistic of 4.741 corresponding to a *p*-value of 0.093.

4. Discussion

This matched case-control study examined the effect of anticoagulant treatment on severity and outcome of SAH. The prevalence of SAH in patients on anticoagulants is low and constituted around two and a half percent of all SAH patients congruous with population-wide prevalence of anticoagulant intake. Prior intake of DOAC or VKA was not associated with more severe SAH, or a higher risk of unfavorable outcome. Although we have investigated an overall large cohort of SAH patients, the number of patients on anticoagulation is low, which might distort statistical analyses. Additionally, it is noteworthy that we assessed a cohort of only hospitalized patients and cannot exclude the possibility of a higher out-of-hospital death rate for SAH patients using DOAC or VKA.

A higher proportion of patients on DOAC required mechanical ventilation and experienced systemic infections. The main aim of the matching procedure was to correct for comorbidities associated with anticoagulant use and higher age. Patients with an indication for continuous oral anticoagulant based on vascular- or heart disease tend to be older and have higher rates of cardiovascular risk factors. Instead of correcting for each individual factor (which constitutes a non-exhaustive list), we only corrected for age. This could mean there is still a higher degree of "baseline comorbidity" in the coagulant groups, which is not corrected for. This could explain an increased propensity towards infections in patients on prior anticoagulant treatment. However, it does not explain why this effect was only apparent in DOAC patients.

Hypercoagulability plays a role in the pathogenesis of DCI and microthrombus formation has been observed in in vivo animal SAH models [31,32]. Moreover, there exists observational efficacy of heparin anticoagulation in clinical use to prevent DCI [33]. The results of the Aneurysmal Subarachnoid Hemorrhage Trial RandOmizing Heparin (ASTROH)-trial are highly anticipated [34]. An additional residual dysfunctional coagulation in the subacute phase could prove protective against DCI by mitigating microthrombosis formation. In our comparison to matched controls, the rate of DCI was similar in patients on prior anticoagulant treatment. The subgroups of anticoagulated patients proved too small to focus analyses on DCI here. However, as our understanding of dysfunctional coagulation microvascular hypercoagulability improves, the potentially beneficial side effects of iatrogenic anticoagulation may become clearer.

Approximately two percent of the general population in Western countries is currently on VKA [35]. Mainly driven by population aging, the use of anticoagulants for prevention of stroke and venous thromboembolisms will only continue rising. Unfortunately, this has been paralleled by an increase in anticoagulant-related ICH [36]. As evidence of safety and effectiveness accumulates, new oral anticoagulants will probably supersede VKA for most indications [37]. Although ICH has not been an endpoint in randomized trials comparing DOAC with warfarin [1–4], observational data suggests DOAC-associated ICH presents with smaller bleeding volumes and lower hematoma expansion rates [38–40]. Along with a shorter half-life, the targeting of a single clotting factor by DOAC—opposed to all vitamin K-dependent factors—allows coagulation to recover more swiftly. The successive development of antidotes will further improve the risk profile of anticoagulants in favor of DOAC over VKA.

Increasing accessibility of magnetic resonance imaging has resulted in a higher incidental detection of aneurysms [41–43]. It remains unclear to what extent anticoagulants might be harmful in those patients. Data on the risk of antithrombotics and SAH has been conflicting. Garbe et al. identified phenprocoumon, clopidogrel/ticlopidine, and acetylsalicylic acid intake, to be associated with increased risk of SAH [18]. In contrast, Risselada et al. demonstrated a similar result for VKA but not for platelet aggregation inhibitors [19]. Multiple smaller observational studies refute that the risk of aneurysm rupture is increased in patients receiving systemic anticoagulation [44–46]. Acetylsalicylic acid is currently being tested in the ongoing PROTECT-U trial (Prospective Randomized Open-label Trial to Evaluate risk faCTor management in patients with Unruptured intracranial aneurysms), to address aneurysm wall inflammation, but might be a hazard to the consequences of its anti-aggregating affect [47].

Nonetheless, if rupture occurs, thrombus formation at the rupture site may take more time, presumably leading to more severe bleeding. Our series demonstrates how hospitalized patients on anticoagulants presenting with SAH are not more severely affected than patients without anticoagulant drugs. The opposite effect was demonstrated in a Dutch series of 15 SAH patients on anticoagulant of which 14 were either dead or highly dependent after three months follow-up [48]. The author's explanation for this effect is that the worse clinical condition patients are in from the outset. It is possible that a faster emergency service's response time in densely populated areas (such as the Netherlands) could increase the number of patients reaching medical services alive, but in a worse clinical state.

Our understanding of aneurysm rupture risk is partially based on patients presenting with SAH [49]. This means patients who suffered SAH-induced sudden death are not represented in these statistics. Likewise, the safety of DOAC and anticoagulants in patients with incidental finding of unruptured intracranial aneurysms cannot be resolved solely by looking at SAH patients since anticoagulated patients suffering SAH-related sudden death are not represented. Nevertheless, even in large-scale atrial fibrillation registries of patients on anticoagulants, autopsy-confirmed cause of death—such as aneurysm rupture—has not been a feasible endpoint as autopsy is not consistently performed [50].

5. Limitations

Besides this selection bias, further limitations of this analysis are the retrospective design and the use of statistically constructed control groups. Sample sizes remain small and statistical results must be interpreted with caution. Although our case-matching algorithm corrects for confounding differences in baseline comorbidities associated with patient age and gender, information and potential detection bias cannot be corrected for. Blood concentrations of DOAC, which vary widely between peak and trough levels, were not routinely available. With the availability and increasing affordability of antidotes, the safety issue of anticoagulants will become less relevant when considering risk of hemorrhagic complications after emergent invasive procedures. However, initial hemorrhage severity and the extent of early brain injury it causes is—despite reversals of anticoagulant effect upon hospital submission—responsible for initiating delayed cerebral ischemia. Therefore, studying anticoagulant use in patients suffering subarachnoid hemorrhage will remain relevant.

6. Conclusions

In this two-center observational study of hospitalized aneurysmal SAH patients, iatrogenic coagulopathy, either caused by DOAC or VKA, was not associated with more severe radiological or clinical subarachnoid hemorrhage compared to matched controls. Intake of anticoagulants was not associated with a higher risk of unfavorable outcome. The rate of unfavorable outcome was similar between patients on VKA compared to DOAC. Nevertheless, the safety issue of DOAC and anticoagulants in patients with unruptured intracranial aneurysms cannot be resolved based on this study as out-of-hospital deaths were not accounted for.

Supplementary Materials: The following supporting information can be downloaded at: https://www.mdpi.com/article/10.3390/jcm12041476/s1, Table S1. Results of univariate logistic regression assessing the effect of direct oral anticoagulant (DOAC) or vitamin K antagonist (VKA) treatment on the occurrence of unfavorable outcome (GOS_{1-3}) after 12 months. Table S2. Results of multivariable logistic regression assessing the effect of direct oral anticoagulant (DOAC) or vitamin K antagonist (VKA) treatment on the occurrence of unfavorable outcome (GOS_{1-3}) after 12 months.

Author Contributions: M.V. and R.R. developed the designed this study. M.V., T.R., M.W., C.C.-D., J.S., J.J.V., T.L. and R.R. were involved in the acquisition of data. M.V. and R.R. performed statistical analyses and drafted the manuscript. M.K., A.H., H.C. and M.N. critically reviewed and edited the manuscript. All authors reviewed and approved the final text. All authors have read and agreed to the published version of the manuscript.

Funding: No funding bodies had any involvement in the preparation of this systematic review, or in the decision to submit the paper for publication.

Institutional Review Board Statement: This study was conducted in accordance with the Declaration of Helsinki and approved by the local ethics committee of the Medical Faculty of RWTH Aachen University (EK 062/14) and of the University of Helsinki and Helsinki University Hospital (HUS/125/2018).

Informed Consent Statement: Due to the retrospective nature of the analysis, the need for patient consent was waived by both local institutional research committees.

Data Availability Statement: The date on which the analyses are based can be made available upon reasonable request from qualified researchers by contacting the corresponding author.

Conflicts of Interest: There are no conflict of interest to report.

Abbreviations

aOR	Adjusted odds ratio
CI	Confidence interval
CT	Computed tomography
DCI	Delayed cerebral ischemia
DOAC	Direct oral anticoagulant
GOS	Glasgow outcome scale
ICH	Intracerebral hemorrhage
ICP	Intracranial pressure
INR	International normalized ratio
IVH	Intraventricular hemorrhage
IQR	Interquartile range
PCC	Prothrombin complex concentrate
PT	Prothrombin time
SAH	Aneurysmal subarachnoid hemorrhage
VKA	Vitamin K antagonist
WFNS	World Federation of Neurological Surgeons

References

1. Connolly, S.J.; Ezekowitz, M.D.; Yusuf, S.; Eikelboom, J.; Oldgren, J.; Parekh, A.; Pogue, J.; Reilly, P.A.; Themeles, E.; Varrone, J.; et al. Dabigatran versus warfarin in patients with atrial fibrillation. *N. Engl. J. Med.* **2009**, *361*, 1139–1151. [CrossRef] [PubMed]
2. Giugliano, R.P.; Ruff, C.T.; Braunwald, E.; Murphy, S.A.; Wiviott, S.D.; Halperin, J.L.; Waldo, A.L.; Ezekowitz, M.D.; Weitz, J.I.; Špinar, J.; et al. Edoxaban versus warfarin in patients with atrial fibrillation. *N. Engl. J. Med.* **2013**, *369*, 2093–2104. [CrossRef] [PubMed]
3. Granger, C.B.; Alexander, J.H.; McMurray, J.J.; Lopes, R.D.; Hylek, E.M.; Hanna, M.; Al-Khalidi, H.R.; Ansell, J.; Atar, D.; Avezum, A.; et al. Apixaban versus warfarin in patients with atrial fibrillation. *N. Engl. J. Med.* **2011**, *365*, 981–992. [CrossRef]
4. Patel, M.R.; Mahaffey, K.W.; Garg, J.; Pan, G.; Singer, D.E.; Hacke, W.; Breithardt, G.; Halperin, J.L.; Hankey, G.J.; Piccini, J.P.; et al. Rivaroxaban versus warfarin in nonvalvular atrial fibrillation. *N. Engl. J. Med.* **2011**, *365*, 883–891. [CrossRef] [PubMed]
5. Raval, A.N.; Cigarroa, J.E.; Chung, M.K.; Diaz-Sandoval, L.J.; Diercks, D.; Piccini, J.P.; Jung, H.S.; Washam, J.B.; Welch, B.G.; Zazulia, A.R.; et al. Management of patients on non-vitamin k antagonist oral anticoagulants in the acute care and periprocedural setting: A scientific statement from the american heart association. *Circulation* **2017**, *135*, e604–e633. [CrossRef]
6. Chan, N.; Sobieraj-Teague, M.; Eikelboom, J.W. Direct oral anticoagulants: Evidence and unresolved issues. *Lancet* **2020**, *396*, 1767–1776. [CrossRef]
7. Mekaj, Y.H.; Mekaj, A.Y.; Duci, S.B.; Miftari, E.I. New oral anticoagulants: Their advantages and disadvantages compared with vitamin K antagonists in the prevention and treatment of patients with thromboembolic events. *Ther. Clin. Risk Manag.* **2015**, *11*, 967–977. [CrossRef]
8. Croci, D.M.; Kamenova, M.; Guzman, R.; Mariani, L.; Soleman, J. Novel oral anticoagulants in patients undergoing cranial surgery. *World Neurosurg.* **2017**, *105*, 841–848. [CrossRef]
9. Pollack, C.V., Jr.; Reilly, P.A.; Eikelboom, J.; Glund, S.; Verhamme, P.; Bernstein, R.A.; Dubiel, R.; Huisman, M.V.; Hylek, E.M.; Kamphuisen, P.W.; et al. Idarucizumab for dabigatran reversal. *N. Engl. J. Med.* **2015**, *373*, 511–520. [CrossRef]
10. Ansell, J.; Laulicht, B.E.; Bakhru, S.H.; Burnett, A.; Jiang, X.; Chen, L.; Baker, C.; Villano, S.; Steiner, S. Ciraparantag, an anticoagulant reversal drug: Mechanism of action, pharmacokinetics, and reversal of anticoagulants. *Blood* **2021**, *137*, 115–125. [CrossRef]
11. Siegal, D.M.; Curnutte, J.T.; Connolly, S.J.; Lu, G.; Conley, P.B.; Wiens, B.L.; Mathur, V.S.; Castillo, J.; Bronson, M.D.; Leeds, J.M.; et al. Andexanet alfa for the reversal of factor xa inhibitor activity. *N. Engl. J. Med.* **2015**, *373*, 2413–2424. [CrossRef] [PubMed]
12. Claassen, J.; Park, S. Spontaneous subarachnoid haemorrhage. *Lancet* **2022**, *400*, 846–862. [CrossRef] [PubMed]
13. Rautalin, I.; Korja, M. Transient intracranial circulatory arrest evidenced at the time of intracranial aneurysm rupture: Case report. *Neurocrit. Care* **2021**, *34*, 340–342. [CrossRef] [PubMed]
14. Huang, J.; van Gelder, J.M. The probability of sudden death from rupture of intracranial aneurysms: A meta-analysis. *Neurosurgery* **2002**, *51*, 1101–1105, discussion 1105–1107. [CrossRef] [PubMed]
15. Swieringa, F.; Spronk, H.M.H.; Heemskerk, J.W.M.; van der Meijden, P.E.J. Integrating platelet and coagulation activation in fibrin clot formation. *Res. Pract. Thromb. Haemost.* **2018**, *2*, 450–460. [CrossRef] [PubMed]

16. Naidech, A.M.; Janjua, N.; Kreiter, K.T.; Ostapkovich, N.D.; Fitzsimmons, B.F.; Parra, A.; Commichau, C.; Connolly, E.S.; Mayer, S.A. Predictors and impact of aneurysm rebleeding after subarachnoid hemorrhage. *Arch Neurol.* **2005**, *62*, 410–416. [CrossRef] [PubMed]
17. Tang, C.; Zhang, T.S.; Zhou, L.F. Risk factors for rebleeding of aneurysmal subarachnoid hemorrhage: A meta-analysis. *PLoS ONE* **2014**, *9*, e99536. [CrossRef]
18. Garbe, E.; Kreisel, S.H.; Behr, S. Risk of subarachnoid hemorrhage and early case fatality associated with outpatient antithrombotic drug use. *Stroke* **2013**, *44*, 2422–2426. [CrossRef]
19. Risselada, R.; Straatman, H.; van Kooten, F.; Dippel, D.W.; van der Lugt, A.; Niessen, W.J.; Firouzian, A.; Herings, R.M.; Sturkenboom, M.C. Platelet aggregation inhibitors, vitamin K antagonists and risk of subarachnoid hemorrhage. *J. Thromb. Haemost.* **2011**, *9*, 517–523. [CrossRef]
20. Witt, D.M.; Nieuwlaat, R.; Clark, N.P.; Ansell, J.; Holbrook, A.; Skov, J.; Shehab, N.; Mock, J.; Myers, T.; Dentali, F.; et al. American society of hematology 2018 guidelines for management of venous thromboembolism: Optimal management of anticoagulation therapy. *Blood Adv.* **2018**, *2*, 3257–3291. [CrossRef]
21. Cuker, A.; Burnett, A.; Triller, D.; Crowther, M.; Ansell, J.; Van Cott, E.M.; Wirth, D.; Kaatz, S. Reversal of direct oral anticoagulants: Guidance from the anticoagulation forum. *Am. J. Hematol.* **2019**, *94*, 697–709. [CrossRef] [PubMed]
22. Piran, S.; Khatib, R.; Schulman, S.; Majeed, A.; Holbrook, A.; Witt, D.M.; Wiercioch, W.; Schünemann, H.J.; Nieuwlaat, R. Management of direct factor xa inhibitor-related major bleeding with prothrombin complex concentrate: A meta-analysis. *Blood Adv.* **2019**, *3*, 158–167. [CrossRef] [PubMed]
23. Virta, J.J.; Satopää, J.; Luostarinen, T.; Raj, R. One-year outcome after aneurysmal subarachnoid hemorrhage in elderly patients. *World Neurosurg.* **2020**, *143*, e334–e343. [CrossRef] [PubMed]
24. Veldeman, M.; Albanna, W.; Weiss, M.; Conzen, C.; Schmidt, T.P.; Schulze-Steinen, H.; Wiesmann, M.; Clusmann, H.; Schubert, G.A. Invasive neuromonitoring with an extended definition of delayed cerebral ischemia is associated with improved outcome after poor-grade subarachnoid hemorrhage. *J. Neurosurg.* **2020**, *134*, 1527–1534. [CrossRef] [PubMed]
25. Frontera, J.A.; Claassen, J.; Schmidt, J.M.; Wartenberg, K.E.; Temes, R.; Connolly, E.S., Jr.; MacDonald, R.L.; Mayer, S.A. Prediction of symptomatic vasospasm after subarachnoid hemorrhage: The modified fisher scale. *Neurosurgery* **2006**, *59*, 21–27. discussion 21–27. [CrossRef]
26. Rosen, D.S.; Macdonald, R.L. Subarachnoid hemorrhage grading scales: A systematic review. *Neurocrit. Care* **2005**, *2*, 110–118. [CrossRef]
27. Jennett, B.; Bond, M. Assessment of outcome after severe brain damage. *Lancet* **1975**, *1*, 480–484. [CrossRef]
28. Vergouwen, M.D.; Vermeulen, M.; van Gijn, J.; Rinkel, G.J.; Wijdicks, E.F.; Muizelaar, J.P.; Mendelow, A.D.; Juvela, S.; Yonas, H.; Terbrugge, K.G.; et al. Definition of delayed cerebral ischemia after aneurysmal subarachnoid hemorrhage as an outcome event in clinical trials and observational studies: Proposal of a multidisciplinary research group. *Stroke* **2010**, *41*, 2391–2395. [CrossRef]
29. Schmidt, T.P.; Weiss, M.; Hoellig, A.; Nikoubashman, O.; Schulze-Steinen, H.; Albanna, W.; Clusmann, H.; Schubert, G.A.; Veldeman, M. Revisiting the timeline of delayed cerebral ischemia after aneurysmal subarachnoid hemorrhage: Toward a temporal risk profile. *Neurocrit. Care* **2022**, *37*, 735–743. [CrossRef]
30. Levy, M.M.; Fink, M.P.; Marshall, J.C.; Abraham, E.; Angus, D.; Cook, D.; Cohen, J.; Opal, S.M.; Vincent, J.L.; Ramsay, G. 2001 sccm/esicm/accp/ats/sis international sepsis definitions conference. *Crit Care Med.* **2003**, *31*, 1250–1256. [CrossRef]
31. Ye, F.; Keep, R.F.; Hua, Y.; Garton, H.J.; Xi, G. Acute micro-thrombosis after subarachnoid hemorrhage: A new therapeutic target? *J. Cereb. Blood Flow Metab.* **2021**, *41*, 2470–2472. [CrossRef]
32. Dienel, A.; Ammassam Veettil, R.; Hong, S.H.; Matsumura, K.; Kumar, T.P.; Yan, Y.; Blackburn, S.L.; Ballester, L.Y.; Marrelli, S.P.; McCullough, L.D.; et al. Microthrombi correlates with infarction and delayed neurological deficits after subarachnoid hemorrhage in mice. *Stroke* **2020**, *51*, 2249–2254. [CrossRef] [PubMed]
33. Kole, M.J.; Wessell, A.P.; Ugiliweneza, B.; Cannarsa, G.J.; Fortuny, E.; Stokum, J.A.; Shea, P.; Chryssikos, T.; Khattar, N.K.; Crabill, G.A.; et al. Low-dose intravenous heparin infusion after aneurysmal subarachnoid hemorrhage is associated with decreased risk of delayed neurological deficit and cerebral infarction. *Neurosurgery* **2021**, *88*, 523–530. [CrossRef]
34. James, R.F. Aneurysmal Subarachnoid Hemorrhage Trial Randomizing Heparin (Astroh). 2015. Available online: https://clinicaltrials.gov/ct2/show/NCT02501434 (accessed on 5 January 2023).
35. Afzal, S.; Zaidi, S.T.R.; Merchant, H.A.; Babar, Z.U.; Hasan, S.S. Prescribing trends of oral anticoagulants in England over the last decade: A focus on new and old drugs and adverse events reporting. *J. Thromb. Thrombolysis* **2021**, *52*, 646–653. [CrossRef]
36. Flaherty, M.L.; Kissela, B.; Woo, D.; Kleindorfer, D.; Alwell, K.; Sekar, P.; Moomaw, C.J.; Haverbusch, M.; Broderick, J.P. The increasing incidence of anticoagulant-associated intracerebral hemorrhage. *Neurology* **2007**, *68*, 116–121. [CrossRef] [PubMed]
37. Zirlik, A.; Bode, C. Vitamin K antagonists: Relative strengths and weaknesses vs. Direct oral anticoagulants for stroke prevention in patients with atrial fibrillation. *J. Thromb. Thrombolysis* **2017**, *43*, 365–379. [CrossRef] [PubMed]
38. Foerch, C.; Lo, E.H.; van Leyen, K.; Lauer, A.; Schaefer, J.H. Intracerebral hemorrhage formation under direct oral anticoagulants. *Stroke* **2019**, *50*, 1034–1042. [CrossRef] [PubMed]
39. Inohara, T.; Xian, Y.; Liang, L.; Matsouaka, R.A.; Saver, J.L.; Smith, E.E.; Schwamm, L.H.; Reeves, M.J.; Hernandez, A.F.; Bhatt, D.L.; et al. Association of intracerebral hemorrhage among patients taking non-vitamin k antagonist vs vitamin k antagonist oral anticoagulants with in-hospital mortality. *JAMA* **2018**, *319*, 463–473. [CrossRef] [PubMed]

40. Kurogi, R.; Nishimura, K.; Nakai, M.; Kada, A.; Kamitani, S.; Nakagawara, J.; Toyoda, K.; Ogasawara, K.; Ono, J.; Shiokawa, Y.; et al. Comparing intracerebral hemorrhages associated with direct oral anticoagulants or warfarin. *Neurology* **2018**, *90*, e1143–e1149. [CrossRef]
41. Vlak, M.H.; Algra, A.; Brandenburg, R.; Rinkel, G.J. Prevalence of unruptured intracranial aneurysms, with emphasis on sex, age, comorbidity, country, and time period: A systematic review and meta-analysis. *Lancet Neurol.* **2011**, *10*, 626–636. [CrossRef]
42. Schievink, W.I. Intracranial aneurysms. *N. Engl. J. Med.* **1997**, *336*, 28–40. [CrossRef] [PubMed]
43. Lawton, M.T.; Vates, G.E. Subarachnoid hemorrhage. *N. Engl. J. Med.* **2017**, *377*, 257–266. [CrossRef] [PubMed]
44. Tarlov, N.; Norbash, A.M.; Nguyen, T.N. The safety of anticoagulation in patients with intracranial aneurysms. *J. Neurointerv. Surg.* **2013**, *5*, 405–409. [CrossRef] [PubMed]
45. Shono, Y.; Sugimori, H.; Matsuo, R.; Fukushima, Y.; Wakisaka, Y.; Kuroda, J.; Ago, T.; Kamouchi, M.; Kitazono, T. Safety of antithrombotic therapy for patients with acute ischemic stroke harboring unruptured intracranial aneurysm. *Int. J. Stroke* **2018**, *13*, 734–742. [CrossRef]
46. Olsen, M.; Johansen, M.B.; Christensen, S.; Sørensen, H.T. Use of vitamin K antagonists and risk of subarachnoid haemorrhage: A population-based case-control study. *Eur. J. Intern. Med.* **2010**, *21*, 297–300. [CrossRef]
47. Vergouwen, M.D.; Rinkel, G.J.; Algra, A.; Fiehler, J.; Steinmetz, H.; Vajkoczy, P.; Rutten, F.H.; Luntz, S.; Hänggi, D.; Etminan, N. Prospective Randomized open-label Trial to evaluate risk factor management in patients with unruptured intracranial aneurysms: Study protocol. *Int. J. Stroke* **2018**, *13*, 992–998. [CrossRef]
48. Rinkel, G.J.; Prins, N.E.; Algra, A. Outcome of aneurysmal subarachnoid hemorrhage in patients on anticoagulant treatment. *Stroke* **1997**, *28*, 6–9. [CrossRef]
49. Bijlenga, P.; Gondar, R.; Schilling, S.; Morel, S.; Hirsch, S.; Cuony, J.; Corniola, M.V.; Perren, F.; Rüfenacht, D.; Schaller, K. PHASES score for the management of intracranial aneurysm: A cross-sectional population-based retrospective study. *Stroke* **2017**, *48*, 2105–2112. [CrossRef]
50. Bassand, J.P.; Virdone, S.; Badoz, M.; Verheugt, F.W.A.; Camm, A.J.; Cools, F.; Fox, K.A.A.; Goldhaber, S.Z.; Goto, S.; Haas, S.; et al. Bleeding and related mortality with noacs and vkas in newly diagnosed atrial fibrillation: Results from the garfield-af registry. *Blood Adv.* **2021**, *5*, 1081–1091. [CrossRef]

Disclaimer/Publisher's Note: The statements, opinions and data contained in all publications are solely those of the individual author(s) and contributor(s) and not of MDPI and/or the editor(s). MDPI and/or the editor(s) disclaim responsibility for any injury to people or property resulting from any ideas, methods, instructions or products referred to in the content.

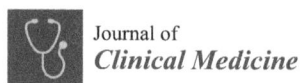 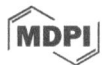

Article

Distal Flow Diversion with Anti-Thrombotically Coated and Bare Metal Low-Profile Flow Diverters—A Comparison

Marie-Sophie Schüngel [1,†], Karl-Titus Hoffmann [2,†], Erik Weber [3], Jens Maybaum [2], Nikolaos Bailis [2], Maximilian Scheer [4], Ulf Nestler [5] and Stefan Schob [1,*]

1. Abteilung für Neuroradiologie, Klinik & Poliklinik für Radiologie, Universitätsklinikum Halle, 06120 Halle (Saale), Germany; marie-sophie.schuengel@uk-halle.de
2. Institut für Neuroradiologie, Universitätsklinikum Leipzig, 04103 Leipzig, Germany
3. Klinik für Anästhesie und Notfallmedizin, Universitätsklinikum Leipzig, 04103 Leipzig, Germany
4. Abteilung für Neurochirurgie, Universitätsklinikum Halle, 06120 Halle (Saale), Germany
5. Klinik und Poliklinik für Neurochirurgie, Universitätsklinikum Leipzig, 04103 Leipzig, Germany
* Correspondence: stefan.schob@uk-halle.de
† These authors contributed equally to this work.

Abstract: Background and purpose: The establishment of low-profile flow diverting stents (FDS), for example, the Silk Vista Baby (SVB) and the p48MW, facilitated endovascular treatment of peripheral cerebral aneurysms. This study therefore aims to compare the performance and outcomes of the SVB with those of the p48MW HPC, with a special focus on hemodynamic aspects of peripheral segments and bifurcations. Materials and methods: The study cohort comprises 108 patients, who were either treated with the SVB or the p48MW HPC between June 2018 and April 2021. Results: Sixty patients received a SVB and forty-eight patients a p48MW HPC. The SVB was used predominantly in the AcomA-complex, and the p48MW HPC in the MCA bifurcation. Immediately after implantation, significant hemodynamic downgrading (OKM A2-A3, B1-B3, C3) was achieved in 60% in the SVB group vs. 75.1% in the p48MW HPC group. At the second follow-up, after an average of 8.8 and 10.9 months, respectively, OKM D1 was observed in 64.4% of the SVB group vs. 27.3% in the p48MW HPC group. Only 1.7% vs. 6.8% of the aneurysms remained morphologically unaltered (OKM A1). Adverse events with persisting neurologic sequalae at last follow-up were largely comparable in both groups (5.0% vs. 4.2%). Conclusion: Immediately after implantation, the p48MW HPC had a more profound hemodynamic impact than the SVB; however, early complete occlusions were achieved in a greater proportion of lesions after implantation of the uncoated SVB.

Keywords: flow diversion; low-profile flow diverter; small cerebral vessels; Silk Vista Baby; p48MW coating

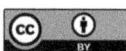

1. Introduction

Flow diversion (FD) has emerged as a reliable, minimally invasive therapeutic concept for cerebral aneurysms [1]. The first FDS were designed and approved exclusively for proximal intracranial aneurysms of the anterior circulation, i.e., the intracranial internal carotid artery from the petrous to the clinoid segment [2]. However, accompanying the success of this approach, challenging indications—for example, post-bifurcational segments of the distal anterior circulation and vertebrobasilar aneurysms—are increasingly considered for flow diversion [3–6].

FDS suitable for the treatment of distal segments of the Circle of Willis require a set of distinct features compared to conventional FDS. For example, catheterization of those segments necessitates well maneuverable, small microcatheters, and, hence, the profile of the corresponding FDS must be comparatively low in order to remain implantable via the latter. Addressing this, low-profile FDS, for instance, the Silk Vista Baby (SVB; Balt, Montmorency, France) and the p48MW (phenox, Bochum, Germany), were developed and are now available for on-label use in small cerebral vessels [7,8]. Both devices are designed for vessel segments ranging from 1.5 mm to 3 mm in diameter and are composed of 48 drawn filled tubing (DFT) strands with an outer nitinol shell and an inner platinum core, the latter providing the required radiopacity for implantation. The SVB is compatible with a 0.017″ microcatheter, whereas the p48MW requires a 0.021″ microcatheter for delivery, but comes with the feature of an independently movable wire (MW), which can be placed 6 cm distal to the target segment for stabilization during implantation in difficult anatomical circumstances [9].

The high surface area coverage of FDS, accounting for approximately 30% of the parent vessel surface, is associated with significant thrombogenicity in vivo [10,11]. Therefore, implantation of FDS requires sufficient inhibition of platelet function in order to avoid thromboembolic events, which is conventionally achieved by administration of dual anti-platelet therapy (DAPT) [12]. The latter, however, may cause critical hemorrhagic complications [13]. A promising approach to the problem of balancing the risk of thromboembolic complications against the risk for hemorrhagic complications associated with FD is the application of surface coating technologies on FDS. One of these biomimicry technologies, for example, uses phosphorycholine, a component of the red blood cell membrane, to cover the surface of the FDS in order to improve its hemocompatibility [14]. In that way, platelets do not adhere to the foreign material of the FDS and the physiological coagulation homeostasis is maintained [10].

Of the currently approved low profile FDS, the p48MW is the only one that is available with an anti-thrombotic hydrophilic polymer coating 'HPC', which distinctly reduces adhesion of platelets [15]. As a consequence, the HPC version of the p48MW allows earlier reduction of DAPT, or even the application of single anti-platelet therapy (SAPT) if the clinical situation demands it [16,17].

Aside from the surface modification of the p48MW HPC the architectures of the SVB and the p48MW are largely comparable. Nevertheless, recent reports indicate that each of the devices may have specific suitability profiles for different cerebrovascular segments, and that time span to aneurysm occlusion post implantation may differ between both devices [8,18]. Therefore, the aim of this study is (a) to report our experiences with both devices for treatment of distally located cerebral aneurysms specifically focusing on their eligibility for different locations and (b) to provide a first comparison of the efficacy, clinical outcomes and angiographic outcomes after implantation of the SVB and the p48MW HPC.

2. Materials and Methods

2.1. Ethics Approval

The retrospective analysis of a prospectively maintained database including patients between June 2018 and April 2021 was approved by the institutional ethics committee (local IRB no AZ 208-15-01062015). Informed consent of each patient regarding the scientific use of radiological and clinical data was obtained in writing either from the patient himself/herself or his/her legal representative.

2.2. Study Design

The prospectively curated institutional database, which includes all endovascular treatments between November 2013 and March 2021, was reviewed to identify all procedures performed employing the Silk Vista Baby or the p48MW HPC, or a combination of both devices. Aneurysms with saccular, blister-like and fusiform morphology were included. Patients with acutely ruptured dissecting aneurysms were not included in this study.

Demographic data, localization, size and morphology of each target lesion, technical and clinical adverse events as well as angiographic follow-up data were collected. Table 1 provides an overview of our patient database.

Table 1. Study population.

	Total	SVB	p48MW HPC
Number of patients	n = 108	n = 60	n = 48
Gender			
Male	33	18	15
Female	75	42	33
Age in years	56 (18–84)	54.1 (18–83)	58.5 (31–84)
Lesion characteristics	n = 114	n = 65	n = 49
Measurements			
Neck width in mm		3.3	3.2
Dome width in mm		4.9	7.4
Dome height in mm		5.4	6.7
Morphology			
Saccular	110	65	45
Fusiform	1	0	1
Blister-like	2	0	2
Dissecting	1	0	1
Localization			
Internal Carotid Artery	21	14	7
Anterior Cerebral Artery	44	37	7
Middle Cerebral Artery	35	8	27
Vertebral Artery	5	4	1
Basilar Artery	8	1	7
Posterior Cerebral Artery	1	1	0
Treatment strategy	n = 108	n = 60	n = 48
Primary	62	30	32
Plug and Pipe	40	27	13
Revision	6	3	3
Procedural aspects			
Total number of implanted devices	128	72	56
Number of implanted SVB			
1	93	51	42
2	11	7	4
3 or more	9	2	2
Adjunctive devices	7	5	2
Anti-platelet regimen			
ASA 100 mg + Ticagrelor 180 mg daily	101	57	44
ASA 100 mg + Clopidogrel 75 mg daily	2	2	0
ASA 100 mg + Prasugrel 10 mg daily	2	1	1
ASA 200–400 mg daily	2	0	2
Prasugrel 10 mg daily	1	0	1
Additional oral anticoagulation	6	4	2

2.3. Anti-Platelet Regimen

DAPT was initiated in all but three patients. The loading doses of 500 mg acetylic salicylic acid (ASA) and either 180 mg ticagrelor (Brilique, AstraZeneca, Hamburg, Germany) or 30 mg prasugrel (Efient, Orifarm, Leverkusen, Germany) or 300 mg clopidogrel (Plavix, 1A Pharma, Holzkirchen, Germany) were administered 24 h prior to the intervention. In emergency cases, however, patients received a bolus of 500 mg ASA intravenously (i.v.) at the beginning of the intervention. In addition, a bolus of body-weight adapted Eptifibatide i.v. (Integrilin, 180 µg/kg; GlaxoSmithKline, Ireland) was given to bridge the duration of the intervention before the second anti-platelet agent was amended orally, immediately after the intervention.

DAPT was then continued as a combination of 100 mg ASA with either ticagrelor 180 mg (given in two single doses of 90 mg 12 h apart) or 10 mg prasugrel or 75 mg clopidogrel daily for at least 12 months, followed by a life-long monotherapy with ASA.

In three cases, a decision was made to keep the patients on SAPT only. The rationale for SAPT in these cases, which demanded a less aggressive inhibition of thrombocyte function, was a preexisting anticoagulation due to cardiologic indication in two patients who remained on ASA only. In the third case, patient anti-platelet therapy with prasugrel only was administered with regards to imminent renal transplantation.

2.4. Endovascular Treatment

All procedures were performed under general anesthesia using a biplane angiography system (Philips AlluraClarity, Best, The Netherlands). An eight French introducer sheath (Terumo radifocus II, Leuven, Belgium) was established via the right common femoral artery and a bolus of 5000 international units of heparin (ratiopharm, Ulm, Germany) was given via the sheath. For triaxial access the guiding catheter was introduced to the respective supra-aortic target vessel with the use of a 5F diagnostic catheter (Cordis TEMPO AQUA) in either Vertebral or Simmons 2 configuration. Either the Neuron Max 088 (6F; Penumbra, Alameda, CA, USA) or the Cerebase (Cerenovus, Irvine, CA, USA) were used as guiding catheters. A 6F Sofia in 115 cm was used as distal access catheter (MicroVention Terumo, Aliso Viejo, CA, USA) in order to increase support for device delivery.

2.4.1. Microcatheters Used for Delivery of the Silk Vista Baby

Depending on the localization of the aneurysm, vessel anatomy and size, different microcatheters were used for implantation of the SVB. In cases of a proximally located aneurysm—i.e., the internal carotid artery (ICA) terminus, the M1 segment of the middle cerebral artery (MCA) or the vertebral artery—the Headway 17 (0.017″; MicroVention Terumo, Aliso Viejo, CA, USA) or the Gama 17 (0.017″; Balt, Montmorency, France) were used. The Headway 17 was initially recommended as delivery catheter; the Gama was specifically designed for the SVB but was released only recently.

In case the target lesion originated from a small peripheral vessel, for example, the pericallosal or callosomarginal artery, or from a challengingly configured complex of the anterior cerebral and anterior communicating arteries, the Excelsior SL10 (0.0165″; Stryker Neurovascular, Cork, Ireland) was used. The latter, however, was only suitable for implantation of the small variants of the SVB with a diameter of 2.25 mm and 2.75 mm, respectively, as described in a prior report [7].

2.4.2. Microcatheters Used for Delivery of the p48MW HPC

The p48MW HPC requires a 0.021″ microcatheter for delivery. In the majority of patients, the Prowler Select Plus (0.021″; Cerenovus, Irvine, CA, USA) was used. However, related to repeated difficulties during catheterization of challengingly curved vessels, the Headway 21 (0.021″; MicroVention Terumo, Aliso Viejo, CA, USA) was tried and then used as a favored microcatheter for p48MW delivery in later interventions.

2.5. Post-Interventional Course and Follow-Up

After the intervention, all patients were transferred to the intensive care unit (ICU) ensuring continuous monitoring for a minimum of 24 h and neurological examination. Non-enhanced cranial computed tomography (CCT) was performed within 24 h post-interventionally in every case.

Routinely, radiography was then performed 4 weeks after FDS implantation for assessment of possible device-induced vasospasm [19]. Angiographic follow-ups were planned at 3, 9 and 24 months after the intervention [20].

3. Results

3.1. Baseline Characteristics

A total of 108 patients (33 men and 75 women; average age of 56.3 years) harboring 114 lesions met the inclusion criteria and were comprised in our analysis. Therefrom, the majority of aneurysms (110/114; 96.5%) were of the saccular side-wall type, 1.8% were blister-like aneurysms and 0.9% were fusiform aneurysms.

The target lesions were distributed as follows: aneurysms were most commonly located in the anterior circulation (100/114; 87.7%). Of them, 21% (21/100) originated from the terminus of the internal carotid artery including the posterior communicating artery (PcomA), 44% (44/100) from the anterior cerebral artery (ACA) starting with the A1-A2 junction also including distal segments, such as the pericallosal artery, and 35% (35/100) from the middle cerebral artery. The remaining lesions (14/114; 12.3%) were located in the posterior circulation. Of those, 35.7% (5/14) arose from the vertebral artery including the PICA orifice, 57.1% (8/14) from the basilar artery, and one aneurysm (7.1%) was located at the posterior cerebral artery.

On average, 1.12 FDS per patient were implanted. In 93 patients a single flow diverter was sufficiently implanted; 11 patients required deployment of two FDS to ensure sufficient treatment of the target lesion. In four cases, however, three or more devices were implanted in telescoping technique.

3.2. Comparison of the SVB and p48MW HPC: Patients and Treatments

More than half of the patients ($n = 60$) were treated with the SVB, the remaining 48 patients were treated with the p48MW HPC. The following differences regarding demographic data and distribution of the aneurysms were observed between the groups: on average, the patients treated with the SVB were younger (54.1 years vs. 58.5 years for the p48MW HPC group) and were more frequently male. The majority of aneurysms in the SVB group originated from the anterior cerebral artery including the pericallosal artery (56.9%). The p48MW HPC group had more than half of the aneurysms in the MCA complex (55.1%). Endovascular treatments in the posterior circulation were more frequently performed using the p48MW HPC. More specifically, 16.3% of the treatments in the p48MW HPC group were performed in the posterior circulation, whereas only 9.2% in the SVB group had posterior circulation aneurysms. Table 2 provides an overview of the anatomical distribution of the respective aneurysms.

Table 2. Overview of the treated lesions.

	SVB	p48MW HPC
Total of treated lesions	$n = 65$	$n = 49$
A1-A2-Acom	29	6
Pericallosal Artery	8	1
M1 Segment	2	5
MCA Bifurcation/M2	6	22
Carotid T	1	1
ICA	9	5
Posterior Communicating Artery	4	1
V4 Segment/PICA Orifice	4	1
PCA/SCA incl. BA	2	7
Assessment of aneurysm occlusion		
Immediately after flow diversion	$n = 65$	$n = 48$ *
OKM A1	26	12
OKM A2-A3	31	33
OKM B	7	3

Table 2. Cont.

	SVB	p48MW HPC
OKM C	1	0
OKM D	0	0
Last available angiographic follow-up	n = 59	n = 44
OKM A1	1	3
OKM A2–A3	3	5
OKM B	11	17
OKM C	5	5
OKM D	38	14
Technical adverse events	n = 6	n = 8
Retraction/Foreshortening/Dislocation	6	5
Insufficient opening	0	2
Secondary FDS kinking	0	1
Peri-interventional adverse events	n = 4	n = 1
Delay in distal perfusion	1	1
Thrombus formation/vessel occlusion	2	0
Extravasate	1	0
Clinical adverse events	n = 8	n = 8
Clinical manifest vasospasm/TIA	2	3
Symptomatic progredience in aneurysm size	1	0
Inflammation of aneurysm wall	0	1
Stent occlusion	2	1
Infarction	2	0
Intracerebral or subarachnoid hemorrhage	1	1
Other hemorrhage	0	1
Clinically manifest adverse events at last follow-up	3	2

* One case of a long-range dissecting aneurysm of the distal vertebral artery was not included for the assessment of the aneurysm occlusion rates using the O'Kelly–Marotta grading scale.

The lesion morphology also differed between the two groups. All patients who were treated with the SVB suffered from saccular shaped side-wall aneurysms. In the p48MW HPC group, in contrast, a slightly smaller proportion (91.8%) of the patients were suffering from saccular side-wall aneurysms. A total of 4.1% had blister-like aneurysms and, respectively, 2.1% had fusiform aneurysms.

Flow diversion was successful in all cases. However, supplementary devices were required in 8.3% (5/60 in the SVB group) vs. 4.2% (2/48 in the p48MW HPC group) of the patients to ensure sufficient treatment of the target lesion. In a total of three patients, who presented with exceptionally large-sized aneurysms, additional coils were loosely deployed within the aneurysm dome prior to FDS implantation aiming to facilitate thrombus formation.

In two cases implantation of further FDS was required. These were related to a patient suffering from a large, broad-based aneurysm arising from the right-sided C6 segment of the internal carotid artery, consequently included in both treatment groups. Due to distal retraction of the initially implanted SILK + (Balt, Montmorency, France) and distinctly varying diameters of the vessel segments proximal and distal to the target lesion, supplementary FDS including the SVB as well as the p48MW HPC were implanted in plug and pipe technique to sufficiently cover the aneurysm neck. In another patient presenting with a wide-necked aneurysm arising from the anterior communicating artery, flow-T stenting was considered as the most promising treatment approach [21]. Therefore, the bilateral distal A2 segments were probated. Firstly, the SVB was deployed into the contralateral A2 segment, proximally ending at the level of the aneurysm neck. Coils were implanted in the bifurcation aneurysm. The LEO+ Baby stent (Balt, Montmorency, France) was then implanted into the ipsilateral A1–A2 junction. One patient presented with a saccular aneurysm of the basilar artery (BA) tip and an additional endoluminal stenosis of the BA segment proximal to the aneurysm with hemodynamic impact to the downstream territory. Therefore, a balloon-expandable coronary stent (REBEL, Boston Scientific) was implanted beyond the SVB to achieve a functionally satisfying result.

3.3. Adverse Events

3.3.1. Technical Challenges

In the SVB group, retraction or distinct foreshortening of the implanted device immediately after deployment occurred in five patients (8.3%). In all these cases, implantation of a second SVB in telescoping technique was required. Device shortenings were either the result of undersizing the implant or of significant elongation and the tortuous course of the target vessel. However, none of the patients suffered from clinical sequelae related to the initial technical obstacles. In one further patient suffering from an incidental aneurysm arising from the origin of the posterior communicating artery, the SVB was successfully implanted into the ipsilateral ICA. However, distal device shortening was detected at the second angiographic follow-up five months post-intervention resulting in insufficient coverage of the aneurysm neck. Re-treatment was necessary and then performed using a second-generation Pipeline Embolization Device (PED2; Medtronic, Covidien, Minneapolis, MN, USA).

In patients treated with the p48MW HPC, technical adverse events were observed in seven cases (14.6%). In two, the FDS showed insufficient opening with incomplete wall apposition immediately after deployment. Additional angioplasty using a compliant balloon (Scepter C; MicroVention Terumo, Aliso Viejo, CA, USA) was performed and resolved the issue in both cases. Dislocation of the p48MW HPC during implantation occurred in three patients. Therefrom, in two patients, the FDS was completely recaptured, removed and substituted by another p48MW HPC. In the third patient, the p48MW HPC dislocated immediately after deployment and required implantation of two further FDS in plug and pipe technique to ensure adequate coverage of the aneurysm neck. Deployment of the second device was uneventful in each case. In the two remaining patients, the FDS had markedly shortened immediately after implantation as a consequence of tortuous segmental anatomy. However, there were no clinical manifestations associated with these technical events.

In one patient who suffered from a fusiform aneurysm of the basilar artery tip, one p48MW was implanted using the proximal P1 segment of the right posterior cerebral artery as distal landing zone and the distal third of the basilar artery as proximal landing zone. Although the patient did not suffer from any neurological deficits at any time, the patient's first angiographic follow-up five months after treatment revealed a significant stenosis of the treated segment at the PCA orifice. In order to prevent ischemic complications, balloon angioplasty was performed, but did not result in significant improvement of the lesion. Therefore, a coronary stent (Rebel; Boston Scientific, Maple Grove, MN, USA) was implanted and achieved permanent reconstruction of the vessel. The patient remained clinically asymptomatic.

3.3.2. Peri-Interventional Adverse Events

In the SVB group four adverse events (6.7%) occurred; three were ischemic and one was hemorrhagic. Ischemic events included transient side branch occlusion and distinctly delayed perfusion of the territory distal to the FDS as well as thrombus formation between two implanted FDS. In all cases, an intravenous bolus of body-weight adapted Eptifibatide (GlaxoSmithKline, Ireland) was administered immediately, followed by continuous infusion for 24 h. In the case of thrombus formation between the not completely adapted layers of two telescopically implanted flow diverter stents, additional angioplasty (Scepter C) was performed and resulted in improved alignment of the FDS with each other and with the vessel wall. In another patient exhibiting two incidental aneurysms of the paraophthalmic ICA, the injection after microcatheter probation revealed contrast extravasation from the aneurysm sack. The SVB was rapidly deployed sufficiently covering the target segment. In the control injection, the extravasation had stopped. Minor subarachnoid hemorrhage

(SAH) was revealed by the control cCT the day after the intervention; however, the patient did not suffer from any clinical sequelae.

In the p48MW HPC group, a distinct delay in perfusion of the covered side branch immediately after FDS implantation was observed in one case (2.1%). In order to prevent any ischemic events, a bolus of Eptifibatide was administered as described above. Perfusion normalized completely and the patient did not show any neurological sequelae post intervention.

3.3.3. Clinical Adverse Events

The SVB group

Adverse events in the SVB group causing clinically relevant sequelae occurred in eight of sixty patients (13.3%). However, the majority of patients recovered completely. At the last clinical follow-up, only three patients (5.0%) still presented with neurological impairment. Additionally, no treatment-related deaths within were observed during the study period.

In two of the eight patients, transient cerebral ischemia manifested clinically after stent occlusion in the early post-interventional course, within 72 h after the treatment. Both received a bolus of body-weight adapted Eptifibatide i.v. In one patient, the thrombus resolved completely together with the patient's neurologic symptoms comprising an acute partial hemiparesis. In the second patient, the SVB remained occluded despite rescue therapy with intravenous Eptifibatide; however, the network of leptomeningeal collaterals connecting the ACA- and MCA periphery maintained perfusion of the affected territory in a retrograde fashion. At the last clinical follow-up, the patient showed good recovery and presented only subtle residual speech disturbances (mRS1).

Subacute device-induced vasospasm with temporary clinical manifestations, a phenomenon reported only recently [19], manifested in two patients without permanent neurological deficits.

Ischemic infarction in the early post-interventional course after FDS implantation was observed in two individuals. The first of these patients had mild aphasia after endovascular treatment of an aneurysm arising from the left-hand side pericallosal artery. Control cCT revealed areas of infarction in the unilateral territory of the ACA and a small part of the anterior third of the MCA territory. However, the neurologic deficits resolved completely within few days, prior to discharge from the hospital. In the other patient, revision treatment of a relapsed AcomA-aneurysm after coiling was performed by implanting the FDS in crossover-technique from the left-hand side A1 segment into the right-hand side A2 segment. Despite technical successful deployment, the control injection 15 min after implantation revealed a delayed perfusion of the covered left-sided A2 segment. Eptifibatide was administered immediately, significantly improving the perfusion of the downstream ACA territory. Still, the patient presented with severe hypodynamic delirium six hours after the intervention. Subsequently initiated cCT revealed partial bilateral infarctions of the ACA- and MCA territories, most likely related to peri-interventional microembolism in the course of the extended procedure time. Despite that, the patient showed good recovery (mRS1) until last clinical follow-up and only presented residual transient speech disturbance.

One case of acute frontobasal parenchymal hemorrhage causing subfalcine herniation occurred 12 h after FDS implantation demanding immediate craniotomy. Despite this major complication, the patient showed an almost complete recovery a few months later, only presenting with mild residual difficulties in walking at the last clinical follow-up (mRS 2). Another patient exhibiting an unstable, partially thrombosed aneurysm of the left-sided MCA experienced a brachial hemiparesis as a result of increased perifocal edema of the aneurysm after implantation of the SVB. Prophylactic corticosteroids had already been started prior to the intervention, which was then amended by Celecoxib 100 mg (Celebrex, Kohlpharma GmbH, Merzig, Germany) daily. The paresis resolved completely within five days.

The p48MW group

In the p48MW HPC group, clinical impairment post intervention was observed in eight patients (16.6%); however, at the last clinical follow-up, only two (4.2%) still presented residual neurological deficits. Comparable to the SVB, treatment-related mortality did not occur within this group.

Three of these eight patients had hemorrhagic complications. Intracranial hemorrhage in the aftermath of FDS implantation occurred in two cases. One patient who underwent revision treatment after flow diversion of a left vertebral artery (V3-V4) dissecting aneurysm presented with prolonged postoperative recovery together with newly developed anisocoria after extubation despite a technically uneventful intervention. The immediate cCT revealed a remote cerebellar hemorrhage which was surgically evacuated. The other patient, who was treated for a MCA-bifurcation aneurysm, suffered from right-frontal intracerebral hemorrhage within 72 h after endovascular therapy, demanding an external ventricular drainage in the early phase. The third patient developed epistaxis and hematemesis in the early post-interventional course most likely related to a Mallory–Weiss lesion that was exacerbating under DAPT. However, two out of three patients recovered completely from the hemorrhage. Only one kept mild neurologic deficits (mRS1) up to the last available clinical follow-up.

In one patient cerebral ischemia manifested after successful treatment of a MCA bifurcation aneurysm within 24 h after the intervention. Although a body-weight adapted bolus of Eptifibatide was administered immediately, the matters were further complicated by the patient's need for an oral anticoagulation due to a cardiologic indication. After secondary hemorrhagic transformation of the partial MCA infarction, protective hemicraniectomy was required. At the last clinical follow-up, the patient still presented moderate neurological impairment comprising hemiparesis and speech disturbance (mRS3).

Device-induced subacute vasospasm without permanent sequelae manifested in one patient. Two patients experienced minor stroke within four months after implantation of the p48MW HPC manifesting with a transient hemiparesis. MRI revealed subtle embolic infarcts in both patients. Both patients recovered completely during the initial hospital stay. In a patient suffering from a giant basilar artery aneurysm, inflammatory changes of the aneurysm wall with MRI contrast enhancement and perifocal edema caused brain stem affection 18 months after the procedure. Neurological impairment resolved completely after anti-inflammatory therapy with cortisone.

3.4. Angiographic Outcome

3.4.1. Hemodynamic Changes Immediately after Flow Diversion

In the SVB group, the majority of the treated lesions (47.7%) immediately showed a marked delay in aneurysm perfusion (OKM A2-A3). Moreover, in 10.8% the aneurysm dome remained only partially perfused corresponding to OKM B1-B3. In one case (1.5%) of a peripheral MCA aneurysm arising from a small side branch of the superior trunk, a very profound hemodynamic effect was observed with a neck remnant only (OKM C3). However, 40% of the aneurysms did not show any immediate hemodynamic changes (OKM A1).

In the p48MW HPC group, the great majority of the treated lesions (68.8%) showed a prolonged stasis of contrast agent within the aneurysm dome (OKM A2-A3) immediately after implantation of the flow diverting stent. In 6.3% of the cases, the target lesion remained only partially perfused (OKM B1-B3). No observable changes in hemodynamics (OKM A1) were seen in 25% of the treated lesions.

3.4.2. Hemodynamic Changes after the First Angiographic Follow-Up

The first angiographic follow-up after an average of 3.1 months and 3.9 months, respectively, was available in 54 patients (59 aneurysms) of the SVB group and in 43 patients (44 aneurysms) after treatment with the p48MW HPC.

More than half of the aneurysms (52.5%) treated with the SVB were already completely occluded, according to OKM D1. A further 33.9% revealed a distinct decrease in perfusion of the aneurysm dome (OKM B-C), and 8.5% showed delayed perfusion (OKM A2-A3). Only 5.1% of the treated lesions remained morphologically unaltered according to OKM A1.

An exemplary case of successful aneurysm treatment using the SVB low-profile flow diverter is shown in Figure 1.

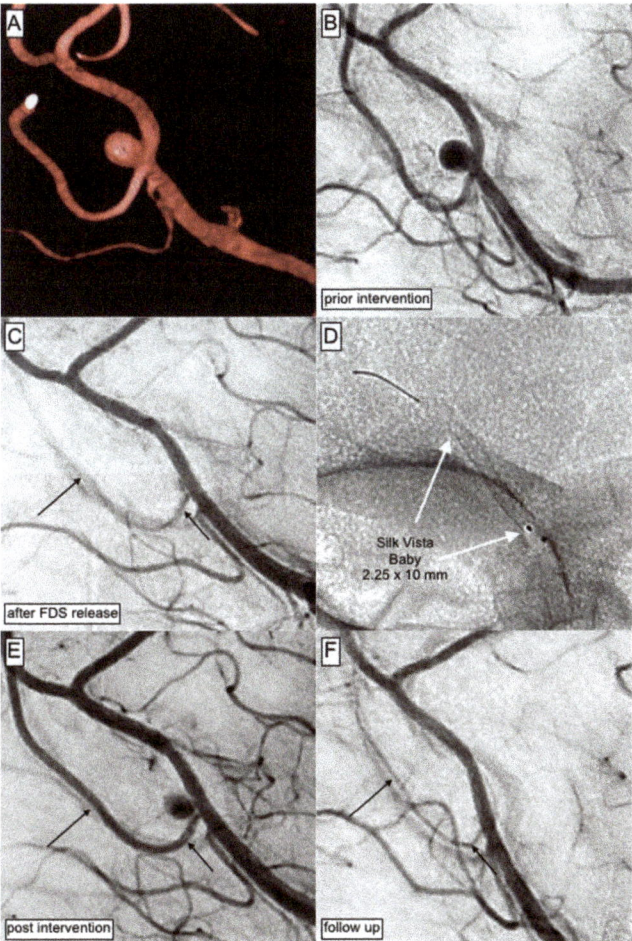

Figure 1. Shows the endovascular therapy of an incidental aneurysm in the distal ACA with the Silk Vista Baby flow diverter. (**A**) The reconstructed 3D angiogram demonstrates a saccular, broad-based aneurysm arising from the left-handed distal ACA at the level of the pericallosal artery. (**B**) Conventional DSA in working projection prior to the FDS implantation. (**C**) The SVB was implanted without any technical obstacles; however, diminished opacification of the covered callosomarginal artery was observed immediately afterwards and required rescue treatment with a GPIIb/IIIa inhibitor. (**D**) Correct position and complete wall adaptation of the implanted device sufficiently covering the aneurysm neck. (**E**) After administration of a body-weight adapted bolus of Eptifibatide intravenously, the control angiogram showed restored perfusion of the covered branch and the downstream territory. In the aftermath of the intervention, the patient did not suffer from neurological deficits. (**F**) At the first angiographic follow-up three months after FDS implantation, the covered segment shows distinct narrowing and the target aneurysm is completely occluded (OKM D1).

Compared to these results, a significantly smaller proportion of aneurysms treated with the p48MW HPC was completely occluded at first follow-up (OKM D1; 22.7%). The vast majority of lesions (52.3%) revealed decline in perfusion and aneurysm size according to OKM B-C.

3.4.3. Hemodynamic Changes at the Second Angiographic Follow-Up

The second follow-up was performed after a mean of 8.8 months and 10.9 months, respectively. The rates of complete aneurysm occlusion (OKM D1) significantly increased in both treatment groups (64.4% vs. 27.3% in the p48MW HPC group). Only 1.7% of the aneurysms after SVB implantation and 6.8% after p48MW HPC treatment still remained morphologically unaltered.

Detailed information concerning the timeline of aneurysm occlusion in the individual cases is given in Table 2.

Figure 2 exposes an exemplary case of aneurysm occlusion following implantation of the p48MW HPC flow diverter.

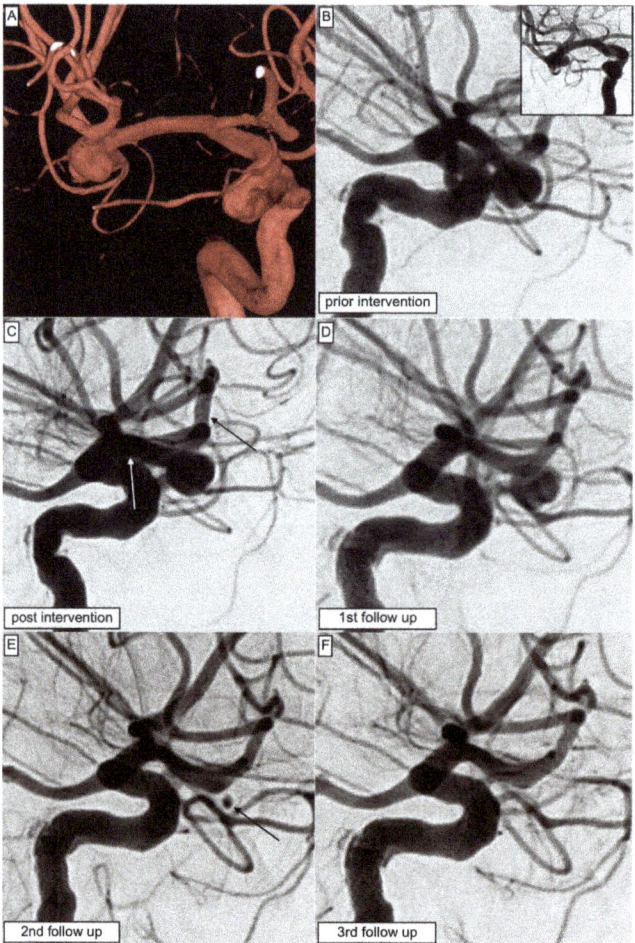

Figure 2. Shows the primary treatment of an irregular-shaped aneurysm arising from the right-hand side MCA trifurcation using the p48MW HPC: (**A**) The reconstructed 3D angiogram demonstrates the broad neck of the aneurysm completely comprising the MCA trifurcation segment. (**B**) Initial

angiogram in working projection prior to the intervention. The posterior–anterior view is presented in the upper right corner. (**C**) After successful implantation of the p48MW HPC with the distal landing zone at the dominant superior trunk. The white arrow indicates the proximal landing zone, and the black arrow shows the distal ending of the FDS. Control injection confirmed the timely perfusion of the complete MCA territory without any delay in perfusion. (**D**) At the first angiographic follow-up, the opacification of the aneurysm remained unaltered (OKM A1); moreover, the side branches do not reveal any significant morphological changes. (**E**) At the second follow-up nine months after the FDS implantation, a significant reduction in aneurysm size with only residual opacification of the aneurysm neck was observed, corresponding to OKM C1. The perfusion of the covered MCA branches remained unaltered. (**F**) At the last available follow-up, 18 months after the treatment, the aneurysm was completely excluded from the intracranial circulation, while the covered M2 branches all remained intact.

4. Discussion

FDS have become a well-established endovascular concept for cerebral aneurysms; however, there is only limited clinical experience with anti-thrombogenic coatings applied to the surface of FDS [8]. Furthermore, differences regarding treatment effects between bare metal (uncoated) and anti-thrombogenically coated FDS in small cerebral vessels have not been systematically investigated. Therefore, our study reviewed treatments with two frequently implanted, structurally comparable low-profile FDS, the SVB representing an uncoated FDS and the p48MW HPC as FDS with an anti-thrombogenic coating.

The architectures of the SVB and the p48MW HPC are similar; both are made of 48 nitinol strands with an inner platinum core. In contrast to the SVB, the p48MW is available with an anti-thrombogenic coating (hydrophilic polymer coating; HPC) that minimizes platelet adhesion together with clot formation in comparison to the uncoated version [22]. The hydrophilic coating was designed to imitate the glycocalyx of the intima of the vessel wall and to prevent inflammation [15]. In situations when dual anti-platelet therapy is not feasible, for example, after acute subarachnoid hemorrhage, the p48MW with HPC modification can be implanted under SAPT [17,23].

Although the structure of both stents is almost identical, the early hemodynamic effect on aneurysm perfusion and the time to definite occlusion differed considerably. More patients treated with the p48MW HPC showed reduced aneurysmal perfusion immediately after stenting (75.1%) compared to the SVB group (60%).

However, the follow-up results showed a diametrically opposed trend: only 27.3% of the aneurysms treated with the p48MW HPC were completely occluded at second follow-up compared to 64.4% completely occluded lesions in the SVB group. This suggests that further variables beyond the mechanical properties of the implants are at least equally important contributors to the therapeutic success.

The time to occlusion of an aneurysm after FDS treatment depends on a number of anatomical, hemodynamic and biological variables. In terms of angioarchitecture and hemodynamics, the magnitude of flow within the parent vessel, wall shear stress, dome to neck ratio, inflow angle, involvement of a bifurcation with or without competitive inflow (for example AcomA-complex vs. MCA-trifurcation) and the distance between aneurysm and parent vessel are known to influence the therapeutic effect after flow diversion [4,24–28]. Aside from that, the process of neointimalization, which biologically depends on disruption of endothelium at the landing zones, local inflammation, activation and binding of platelets to the implanted device together with the subsequent recruitment of circulating endothelial progenitor cells, dictates the timeframe of vascular healing after flow diverter treatment of an artery [29].

Anti-thrombogenic coatings and anti-platelet drugs both interfere with the cellular processes involved in the progress of vascular healing [30]. Since the anti-platelet medication was consistent in our patients, the hydrophilic coating of the p48MW constitutes the only elementary therapeutic difference between the two groups. As HPC inhibits platelet adhesion and activation, we consider the HPC surface modification of the p48MW to be a major factor involved in the longer time to aneurysm occlusion.

So far, meaningful evidence in this regard is scarce. Bhogal et al. demonstrated near-complete neoendothelialization 30 and 180 days after pCONus implantation, independent from the presence or absence of the HPC coating [31]. However, this study differs significantly from our analysis. First, the stent construct of the pCONus adjacent to the vessel wall is made of four wires only and therefore has a distinctly lower surface metal coverage than a FDS [32], requiring only a very small amount of neointima for coverage. Second, ASA and Clopidogrel were administered in Bhogal's study, whereas the standard regimen at our neurovascular center comprised ASA and Ticagrelor.

Both Clopidogrel and Ticagrelor inhibit platelet aggregation via blockage of the P2Y12 receptor that is expressed on the cell surface. Apart from the anti-aggregant effect on platelets, only Ticagrelor is a strong inhibitor of the nucleotide receptor P2Y12, which mediates a variety of further, at this time not completely comprehended, mechanisms. Smooth muscle cells of the vessels and endothelial cells both carry P2Y12 nucleotide receptors. In vitro studies proved the inhibitory effect of P2Y12 nucleotide blockade on endothelial cell proliferation irrespective of the anti-aggregative effects [33]. Improved endothelial function was present after administration of Ticagrelor in patients suffering coronary arterial disease or chronic obstructive pulmonary disease [34]. This effect may be explained by a Ticagrelor-induced decrease in serum levels of the epidermal growth factor (EGF), the latter playing a major role in the genesis of endothelial dysfunction including atherosclerosis and vessel remodeling [35]. Apart from that, inhibition of the transmembrane protein equilibrative nucleoside transporter 1 (ENT1) mediated by ticagrelor has a major impact on the ticagrelor-driven anti-inflammatory effects [36].

As a consequence of the aforementioned, the choice of the second anti-aggregant certainly also influences the efficacy and speed of vascular healing after FDS implantation. However, as the majority of all patients in our study received Ticagrelor, the longer period until aneurysm occlusion in the p48MW HPC group is unlikely to be a consequence of a different DAPT medication scheme.

In our study, the p48MW HPC was preferentially implanted in the MCA (55.1%), whereas the SVB was mostly implanted into the ACA (56.9%). The hemodynamic situation in both territories varies significantly. For example, mean flows and mean velocities are significantly greater in the MCA than the ACA [37].

Furthermore, depending on the symmetry or asymmetry of the AcomA-complex, AcomA-aneurysms have potential inflow from two sources [38–40]. In case of proximal asymmetry, for example, a type 4 complex according to the classification of Krzyżewski and colleagues, where one dominant A1 segment predominantly supplies the ACA territory with only a minor contribution via the hypoplastic contralateral A1, to which it is connected to by an AcomA, the asymmetry actually facilitates aneurysm occlusion after unilateral hemodynamic intervention. More specifically, the flow diverter deployed in the dominant A1-A2 segment reduces ipsilateral inflow to the AcomA, and subsequently, the inflow via the contralateral, hypoplastic A1 becomes equally strong, resulting in a pressure equilibrium within the AcomA, and hence, aneurysm occlusion [4,41].

As a comparable hemodynamic situation with conflicting flows being present within the bifurcation itself does not occur under regular circumstances in the MCA bifurcation, but the M2 branches rather competitively drain blood from the MCA mainstem, so blood flow velocities usually remain stronger after FDS deployment. Therefore, a prolonged time to aneurysm occlusion after p48MW HPC may not only be the result of the anti-thrombotic coating, but also a consequence of the distinct, less favorable hemodynamic situation in the MCA compared to the ACA.

However, in our experience, a longer period between the implantation of a FDS and its complete coverage by neointima does not constitute a disadvantage, especially not when treating incidental aneurysms. When significant terminal branches arising in close proximity to the aneurysm are covered by the FDS for technical reasons, or when the hemodynamic situation in a bi- or trifurcation anatomy with only one inflow source is profoundly altered, the slower occlusion allows for more collateral vessels to develop, the prevention of ischemic events being supported by the DAPT.

In this regard, especially MCA-bifurcation aneurysms as a target for flow diversion are being discussed controversially with conflicting clinical evidence [42]. Cagnazzo et al. found 20% treatment-related complications with half of them having permanent clinical sequelae in an earlier study [43]. Diestro et al. reported 16% thromboembolic complications after FD of the proximal MCA bifurcation in a collective of patients who required retreatment after a failed first surgical or endovascular attempt [44]. Contrary to that, Salem et al. found that MCA-bifurcation aneurysms are treatable with much lower complication rates, the outcomes of their study being comparable to other, well consented FD locations [45]. Cimflova and coworkers contributed their experience with less than 9% significant complications after FD implantation in the MCA distal to the M1 segment [46].

Limitations

The presented results were collected from a single center only, and consequently, are lacking a multicentric comparison and a greater study cohort. Furthermore, the difference regarding the predominant target vessels, namely the MCA for the p48MW HPC vs. the ACA territory for the SVB, represents a relevant bias in our study. Therefore, a prospective investigation with comparable treatment groups for each territory, even for the proximal ACA- and the proximal MCA-bifurcation, is wanted.

5. Conclusions

This study demonstrates a comparable safety profile of both FDS, the SVB and the p48MW HPC, for the endovascular therapy of peripheral intracranial aneurysms with differing early and late therapeutic outcomes when comparing both devices. While the SVB apparently achieved enhanced rates of early complete aneurysm occlusion, this may be influenced by its predominant use in the ACA territory in our study cohort. The rates of early aneurysm occlusion after treatment with the p48MW HPC were lower; however, the FDS was mostly deployed in the MCA territory, encountering different hemodynamic circumstances. With respect to the MCA perforators and the possible risk of thromboembolic events when covering side branches, the anti-thrombogenic coating of the p48MW HPC together with double anti-platelet therapy offers the advantage of prolonged occlusion times allowing for development of collateral vessels.

Author Contributions: Conceptualization, S.S. and M.-S.S.; methodology, J.M. and N.B.; validation, U.N.; formal analysis, M.-S.S. and M.S.; investigation, S.S.; resources, E.W.; data curation, M.-S.S.; writing—original draft preparation, S.S. and M.-S.S.; writing—review and editing, S.S. and K.-T.H.; visualization, S.S.; supervision, S.S.; project administration, S.S. and K.-T.H. All authors have read and agreed to the published version of the manuscript.

Funding: This research received no external funding.

Institutional Review Board Statement: The study was conducted in accordance with the Declaration of Helsinki, and approved by the institutional ethics committee (local IRB no AZ 208-15-0010062015).

Informed Consent Statement: Informed consent was obtained from all subjects involved in the study.

Data Availability Statement: Not applicable.

Conflicts of Interest: The authors declare no conflict of interest.

References

1. Gory, B.; Berge, J.; Bonafé, A.; Pierot, L.; Spelle, L.; Piotin, M.; Biondi, A.; Cognard, C.; Mounayer, C.; Sourour, N.; et al. Flow Diverters for Intracranial Aneurysms: The DIVERSION National Prospective Cohort Study. *Stroke* **2019**, *50*, 3471–3480. [CrossRef] [PubMed]
2. Dmytriw, A.A.; Phan, K.; Moore, J.M.; Pereira, V.M.; Krings, T.; Thomas, A.J. On Flow Diversion: The Changing Landscape of Intracerebral Aneurysm Management. *AJNR Am. J. Neuroradiol.* **2019**, *40*, 591–600. [CrossRef] [PubMed]
3. Kan, P.; Sweid, A.; Srivatsan, A.; Jabbour, P. Expanding Indications for Flow Diverters: Ruptured Aneurysms, Blister Aneurysms, and Dissecting Aneurysms. *Neurosurgery* **2020**, *86* (Suppl. S1), S96–S103. [CrossRef]
4. Schob, S.; Brill, R.; Siebert, E.; Sponza, M.; Schüngel, M.-S.; Wohlgemuth, W.A.; Götz, N.; Mucha, D.; Gopinathan, A.; Scheer, M.; et al. Indirect Flow Diversion for Off-Centered Bifurcation Aneurysms and Distant Small-Vessel Aneurysms, a Retrospective Proof of Concept Study From Five Neurovascular Centers. *Front. Neurol.* **2022**, *12*, 801470. [CrossRef] [PubMed]
5. Maybaum, J.; Henkes, H.; Aguilar-Pérez, M.; Hellstern, V.; Gihr, G.A.; Härtig, W.; Reisberg, A.; Mucha, D.; Schüngel, M.-S.; Brill, R.; et al. Flow Diversion for Reconstruction of Intradural Vertebral Artery Dissecting Aneurysms Causing Subarachnoid Hemorrhage-A Retrospective Study From Four Neurovascular Centers. *Front. Neurol.* **2021**, *12*, 700164. [CrossRef]
6. Hellstern, V.; Aguilar-Pérez, M.; Henkes, E.; Serna-Candel, C.; Wendl, C.; Bäzner, H.; Ganslandt, O.; Henkes, H. Endovascular Treatment of Posterior Circulation Saccular Aneurysms With the p64 Flow Modulation Device: Mid-and Long-Term Results in 54 Aneurysms From a Single Center. *Front. Neurol.* **2021**, *12*, 711863. [CrossRef]
7. Schob, S.; Hoffmann, K.-T.; Richter, C.; Bhogal, P.; Köhlert, K.; Planitzer, U.; Ziganshyna, S.; Lindner, D.; Scherlach, C.; Nestler, U.; et al. Flow diversion beyond the circle of Willis: Endovascular aneurysm treatment in peripheral cerebral arteries employing a novel low-profile flow diverting stent. *J. Neurointerv. Surg.* **2019**, *11*, 1227–1234. [CrossRef]
8. Schob, S.; Kläver, M.; Richter, C.; Scherlach, C.; Maybaum, J.; Mucha, S.; Schüngel, M.-S.; Hoffmann, K.T.; Quaeschling, U. Single-Center Experience With the Bare p48MW Low-Profile Flow Diverter and Its Hydrophilically Covered Version for Treatment of Bifurcation Aneurysms in Distal Segments of the Anterior and Posterior Circulation. *Front. Neurol.* **2020**, *11*, 1050. [CrossRef]
9. Quäschling, U.; Kläver, M.; Richter, C.; Hamerla, G.; Mucha, S.; Scherlach, C.; Maybaum, J.; Hoffmann, K.-T.; Schob, S. Flow diversion in challenging vascular anatomies: The use of low profile stent retrievers for safe and accurate positioning of the microcatheter. *CVIR Endovasc.* **2020**, *3*, 19. [CrossRef]
10. Lenz-Habijan, T.; Bhogal, P.; Peters, M.; Bufe, A.; Moreno, R.M.; Bannewitz, C.; Monstadt, H.; Henkes, H. Hydrophilic Stent Coating Inhibits Platelet Adhesion on Stent Surfaces: Initial Results In Vitro. *Cardiovasc. Interv. Radiol.* **2018**, *41*, 1779–1785. [CrossRef]
11. Girdhar, G.; Li, J.; Kostousov, L.; Wainwright, J.; Chandler, W.L. In-vitro thrombogenicity assessment of flow diversion and aneurysm bridging devices. *J. Thromb. Thrombolysis* **2015**, *40*, 437–443. [CrossRef] [PubMed]
12. Soize, S.; Foussier, C.; Manceau, P.-F.; Litré, C.-F.; Backchine, S.; Gawlitza, M.; Pierot, L. Comparison of two preventive dual antiplatelet regimens for unruptured intracranial aneurysm embolization with flow diverter/disrupter: A matched-cohort study comparing clopidogrel with ticagrelor. *J. Neuroradiol.* **2019**, *46*, 378–383. [CrossRef] [PubMed]
13. Jeong, H.W.; Seo, J.H.; Kim, S.T.; Jung, C.K.; Suh, S.I. Clinical practice guideline for the management of intracranial aneurysms. *Neurointervention* **2014**, *9*, 63–71. [CrossRef] [PubMed]
14. Manning, N.W.; Cheung, A.; Phillips, T.J.; Wenderoth, J.D. Pipeline shield with single antiplatelet therapy in aneurysmal subarachnoid haemorrhage: Multicentre experience. *J. Neurointerv. Surg.* **2019**, *11*, 694–698. [CrossRef] [PubMed]
15. Lenz-Habijan, T.; Brodde, M.; Kehrel, B.E.; Bannewitz, C.; Gromann, K.; Bhogal, P.; Perez, M.A.; Monstadt, H.; Henkes, H. Comparison of the Thrombogenicity of a Bare and Antithrombogenic Coated Flow Diverter in an In Vitro Flow Model. *Cardiovasc. Interv. Radiol.* **2020**, *43*, 140–146. [CrossRef]
16. Bhogal, P.; Bleise, C.; Chudyk, J.; Lylyk, I.; Perez, N.; Henkes, H.; Lylyk, P. The p48_HPC antithrombogenic flow diverter: Initial human experience using single antiplatelet therapy. *J. Int. Med. Res.* **2020**, *48*, 300060519879580. [CrossRef]
17. Aguilar-Perez, M.; Hellstern, V.; AlMatter, M.; Wendl, C.; Bäzner, H.; Ganslandt, O.; Henkes, H. The p48 Flow Modulation Device with Hydrophilic Polymer Coating HPC for the Treatment of Acutely Ruptured Aneurysms: Early Clinical Experience Using Single Antiplatelet Therapy. *Cardiovasc. Interv. Radiol.* **2020**, *43*, 740–748. [CrossRef]
18. Schüngel, M.-S.; Quäschling, U.; Weber, E.; Struck, M.F.; Maybaum, J.; Bailis, N.; Arlt, F.; Richter, C.; Hoffmann, K.-T.; Scherlach, C.; et al. Endovascular Treatment of Intracranial Aneurysms in Small Peripheral Vessel Segments-Efficacy and Intermediate Follow-Up Results of Flow Diversion With the Silk Vista Baby Low-Profile Flow Diverter. *Front. Neurol.* **2021**, *12*, 671915. [CrossRef]
19. Schob, S.; Richter, C.; Lindner, D.; Planitzer, U.; Hamerla, G.; Ziganshyna, S.; Werdehausen, R.; Struck, M.F.; Gaber, K.; Meixensberger, J.; et al. Delayed Stroke after Aneurysm Treatment with Flow Diverters in Small Cerebral Vessels: A Potentially Critical Complication Caused by Subacute Vasospasm. *J. Clin. Med.* **2019**, *8*, 1649. [CrossRef]
20. O'Kelly, C.J.; Krings, T.; Fiorella, D.; Marotta, T.R. A novel grading scale for the angiographic assessment of intracranial aneurysms treated using flow diverting stents. *Interv. Neuroradiol.* **2010**, *16*, 133–137. [CrossRef]
21. Makalanda, H.; Wong, K.; Bhogal, P. Flow-T stenting with the Silk Vista Baby and Baby Leo stents for bifurcation aneurysms—A novel endovascular technique. *Interv. Neuroradiol.* **2020**, *26*, 68–73. [CrossRef]

22. Bhogal, P.; Lenz-Habijan, T.; Bannewitz, C.; Hannes, R.; Monstadt, H.; Brodde, M.; Kehrel, B.; Henkes, H. Thrombogenicity of the p48 and anti-thrombogenic p48 hydrophilic polymer coating low-profile flow diverters in an in vitro human thrombin generation model. *Interv. Neuroradiol.* **2020**, *26*, 488–493. [CrossRef]
23. Schüngel, M.S.; Hoffmann, K.T.; Quäschling, U.; Schob, S. Anterior Cerebral Artery (A1 Segment) Aneurysm: Abandoned Dual Platelet Inhibition Shortly After Endovascular Treatment with a Hydrophilic Polymer-Coated Flow Diverter p48MW HPC; Good Clinical Outcome and Early Aneurysm Occlusion. In *The Aneurysm Casebook*; Henkes, H., Lylyk, P., Ganslandt, O., Eds.; Springer: Cham, Switzerland, 2020. [CrossRef]
24. Fahed, R.; Darsaut, T.E.; Gentric, J.-C.; Farzin, B.; Salazkin, I.; Gevry, G.; Raymond, J. Flow diversion: What can clinicians learn from animal models? *Neuroradiology* **2017**, *59*, 255–261. [CrossRef]
25. Rouchaud, A.; Ramana, C.; Brinjikji, W.; Ding, Y.-H.; Dai, D.; Gunderson, T.; Cebral, J.; Kallmes, D.; Kadirvel, R. Wall Apposition Is a Key Factor for Aneurysm Occlusion after Flow Diversion: A Histologic Evaluation in 41 Rabbits. *AJNR Am. J. Neuroradiol.* **2016**, *37*, 2087–2091. [CrossRef]
26. Nossek, E.; Chalif, D.J.; Levine, M.; Setton, A. Modifying flow in the ACA-ACoA complex: Endovascular treatment option for wide-neck internal carotid artery bifurcation aneurysms. *J. Neurointerv. Surg.* **2015**, *7*, 351–356. [CrossRef]
27. Farnoush, A.; Avolio, A.; Qian, Y. Effect of bifurcation angle configuration and ratio of daughter diameters on hemodynamics of bifurcation aneurysms. *AJNR Am. J. Neuroradiol.* **2013**, *34*, 391–396. [CrossRef]
28. MacLean, M.A.; Huynh, T.J.; Schmidt, M.H.; Pereira, V.M.; Weeks, A. Republished: Competitive flow diversion of multiple P1 aneurysms: Proposed classification. *J. Neurointerv. Surg.* **2020**, *12*, e7. [CrossRef]
29. Ravindran, K.; Casabella, A.M.; Cebral, J.; Brinjikji, W.; Kallmes, D.F.; Kadirvel, R. Mechanism of Action and Biology of Flow Diverters in the Treatment of Intracranial Aneurysms. *Neurosurgery* **2020**, *86* (Suppl. S1), S13–S19. [CrossRef]
30. Cortese, J.; Rasser, C.; Even, G.; Bardet, S.M.; Choqueux, C.; Mesnier, J.; Perrin, M.-L.; Janot, K.; Caroff, J.; Nicoletti, A.; et al. CD31 Mimetic Coating Enhances Flow Diverting Stent Integration into the Arterial Wall Promoting Aneurysm Healing. *Stroke* **2021**, *52*, 677–686. [CrossRef]
31. Bhogal, P.; Lenz-Habijan, T.; Bannewitz, C.; Hannes, R.; Monstadt, H.; Simgen, A.; Mühl-Benninghaus, R.; Reith, W.; Henkes, H. The pCONUS HPC: 30-Day and 180-Day In Vivo Biocompatibility Results. *Cardiovasc. Interv. Radiol.* **2019**, *42*, 1008–1015. [CrossRef]
32. Lubicz, B.; Morais, R.; Alghamdi, F.; Mine, B.; Collignon, L.; Eker, O.F. The pCONus device for the endovascular treatment of wide neck bifurcation aneurysms. *J. Neurointerv. Surg.* **2016**, *8*, 940–944. [CrossRef]
33. Korybalska, K.; Rutkowski, R.; Luczak, J.; Czepulis, N.; Karpinski, K.; Witowski, J. The role of purinergic P2Y12 receptor blockers on the angiogenic properties of endothelial cells: An in vitro study. *J. Physiol. Pharmacol.* **2018**, *69*, 4. [CrossRef]
34. Viecelli Dalla Sega, F.; Fortini, F.; Aquila, G.; Pavasini, R.; Biscaglia, S.; Bernucci, D.; Del Franco, A.; Tonet, E.; Rizzo, P.; Ferrari, R.; et al. Ticagrelor Improves Endothelial Function by Decreasing Circulating Epidermal Growth Factor (EGF). *Front. Physiol.* **2018**, *9*, 337. [CrossRef] [PubMed]
35. Wang, L.; Huang, Z.; Huang, W.; Chen, X.; Shan, P.; Zhong, P.; Khan, Z.; Wang, J.; Fang, Q.; Liang, G.; et al. Inhibition of epidermal growth factor receptor attenuates atherosclerosis via decreasing inflammation and oxidative stress. *Sci. Rep.* **2017**, *8*, 45917. [CrossRef] [PubMed]
36. Nylander, S.; Schulz, R. Effects of P2Y12 receptor antagonists beyond platelet inhibition–comparison of ticagrelor with thienopyridines. *Br. J. Pharmacol.* **2016**, *173*, 1163–1178. [CrossRef]
37. Bammer, R.; Hope, T.A.; Aksoy, M.; Alley, M.T. Time-resolved 3D quantitative flow MRI of the major intracranial vessels: Initial experience and comparative evaluation at 1.5T and 3.0T in combination with parallel imaging. *Magn. Reson. Med.* **2007**, *57*, 127–140. [CrossRef]
38. Castro, M.A.; Putman, C.M.; Sheridan, M.J.; Cebral, J.R. Hemodynamic patterns of anterior communicating artery aneurysms: A possible association with rupture. *AJNR Am. J. Neuroradiol.* **2009**, *30*, 297–302. [CrossRef]
39. Burlakoti, A.; Kumaratilake, J.; Taylor, J.; Henneberg, M. Relationship between cerebral aneurysms and variations in cerebral basal arterial network: A morphometric cross-sectional study in Computed Tomography Angiograms from a neurointerventional unit. *BMJ Open* **2021**, *11*, e051028. [CrossRef]
40. Krzyżewski, R.M.; Tomaszewski, K.A.; Kochana, M.; Kopeć, M.; Klimek-Piotrowska, W.; Walocha, J.A. Anatomical variations of the anterior communicating artery complex: Gender relationship. *Surg. Radiol. Anat.* **2014**, *37*, 81–86. [CrossRef]
41. Colby, G.P.; Bender, M.T.; Lin, L.-M.; Beaty, N.; Huang, J.; Tamargo, R.J.; Coon, A.L. Endovascular flow diversion for treatment of anterior communicating artery region cerebral aneurysms: A single-center cohort of 50 cases. *J. Neurointerv. Surg.* **2017**, *9*, 679–685. [CrossRef]
42. Shah, K.A.; Patsalides, A.; Dehdashti, A.R. Letter: Flow Diversion for Middle Cerebral Artery Aneurysms: An International Cohort Study. *Neurosurgery* **2022**, *90*, e176–e177. [CrossRef]
43. Cagnazzo, F.; Mantilla, D.; Lefevre, P.H.; Dargazanli, C.; Gascou, G.; Costalat, V. Treatment of Middle Cerebral Artery Aneurysms with Flow-Diverter Stents: A Systematic Review and Meta-Analysis. *AJNR Am. J. Neuroradiol.* **2017**, *38*, 2289–2294. [CrossRef]
44. Diestro, J.D.B.; Adeeb, N.; Dibas, M.; Boisseau, W.; Harker, P.; Brinjikji, W.; Xiang, S.; Joyce, E.; Shapiro, M.; Raz, E.; et al. Flow Diversion for Middle Cerebral Artery Aneurysms: An International Cohort Study. *Neurosurgery* **2021**, *89*, 1112–1121. [CrossRef]

45. Salem, M.M.; Khorasanizadeh, M.; Lay, S.V.; Renieri, L.; Kuhn, A.L.; Sweid, A.; Massari, F.; Moore, J.M.; Tjoumakaris, S.I.; Jabbour, P.; et al. Endoluminal flow diverting stents for middle cerebral artery bifurcation aneurysms: Multicenter cohort. *J. Neurointerv. Surg.* **2022**, *14*, 1084–1089. [CrossRef]
46. Cimflova, P.; Özlük, E.; Korkmazer, B.; Ahmadov, R.; Akpek, E.; Kizilkilic, O.; Islak, C.; Kocer, N. Long-term safety and efficacy of distal aneurysm treatment with flow diversion in the M2 segment of the middle cerebral artery and beyond. *J. Neurointerv. Surg.* **2021**, *13*, 631–636. [CrossRef]

Disclaimer/Publisher's Note: The statements, opinions and data contained in all publications are solely those of the individual author(s) and contributor(s) and not of MDPI and/or the editor(s). MDPI and/or the editor(s) disclaim responsibility for any injury to people or property resulting from any ideas, methods, instructions or products referred to in the content.

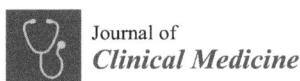

Review

Anti-Inflammatory Drug Therapy in Aneurysmal Subarachnoid Hemorrhage: A Systematic Review and Meta-Analysis of Prospective Randomized and Placebo-Controlled Trials

Johannes Wach *, Martin Vychopen, Agi Güresir and Erdem Güresir

Department of Neurosurgery, University Hospital Leipzig, 04103 Leipzig, Germany;
martin.vychopen@medizin.uni-leipzig.de (M.V.); agi.gueresir@medizin.uni-leipzig.de (A.G.);
erdem.gueresir@medizin.uni-leipzig.de (E.G.)
* Correspondence: johannes.wach@medizin.uni-leipzig.de; Tel.: +49-3419717

Citation: Wach, J.; Vychopen, M.; Güresir, A.; Güresir, E. Anti-Inflammatory Drug Therapy in Aneurysmal Subarachnoid Hemorrhage: A Systematic Review and Meta-Analysis of Prospective Randomized and Placebo-Controlled Trials. *J. Clin. Med.* 2023, 12, 4165. https://doi.org/10.3390/jcm12124165

Academic Editors: Ramazan Jabbarli and Dimitre Staykov

Received: 26 April 2023
Revised: 2 June 2023
Accepted: 17 June 2023
Published: 20 June 2023

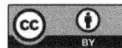

Copyright: © 2023 by the authors. Licensee MDPI, Basel, Switzerland. This article is an open access article distributed under the terms and conditions of the Creative Commons Attribution (CC BY) license (https://creativecommons.org/licenses/by/4.0/).

Abstract: Emerging evidence suggests that neuroinflammation may play a potential role in aneurysmal subarachnoid hemorrhage (aSAH). We aim to analyze the influence of anti-inflammatory therapy on survival and outcome in aSAH. Eligible randomized placebo-controlled prospective trials (RCTs) were searched in PubMed until March 2023. After screening the available studies for inclusion and exclusion criteria, we strictly extracted the main outcome measures. Dichotomous data were determined and extracted by odds ratio (OR) with 95% confidence intervals (CIs). Neurological outcome was graded using the modified Rankin Scale (mRS). We created funnel plots to analyze publication bias. From 967 articles identified during the initial screening, we included 14 RCTs in our meta-analysis. Our results illustrate that anti-inflammatory therapy yields an equivalent probability of survival compared to placebo or conventional management (OR: 0.81, 95% CI: 0.55–1.19, p = 0.28). Generally, anti-inflammatory therapy trended to be associated with a better neurologic outcome (mRS $\leq$ 2) compared to placebo or conventional treatment (OR: 1.48, 95% CI: 0.95–2.32, p = 0.08). Our meta-analysis showed no increased mortality form anti-inflammatory therapy. Anti-inflammatory therapy in aSAH patients tends to improve the neurological outcome. However, multicenter, rigorous, designed, prospective randomized studies are still needed to investigate the effect of fighting inflammation in improving neurological functioning after aSAH.

Keywords: intracranial aneurysm; treatment; subarachnoid hemorrhage; vasospasm; delayed ischemic neurological deficit

1. Introduction

Aneurysmal subarachnoid hemorrhage (aSAH) is a severe neurological disorder that affects 6–9 individuals per 100,000 each year and has a mortality rate of 35% [1]. In recent decades, the incidences of aSAH have decreased globally due to reduced smoking rates and improved management of arterial hypertension [2]. However, mortality and morbidity rates remain high, and survivors often experience poor functional outcomes, with roughly half unable to return to their previous life [3]. Prehospital mortality rates from aSAH are still between 22% and 26% [4]. Additionally, about 35% of aSAH patients suffer from memory disturbances, depression, and reduced quality of life [5–8].

Cerebral vasospasm (CVS) is linked to delayed cerebral ischemia (DCI) and is believed to play a role in unfavorable results following aSAH [9]. In order to enhance outcomes, various rescue therapies are utilized, including the selective intra-arterial infusion of vasodilators, balloon angioplasty, and induced hypertension [3,10]. However, the underlying pathophysiological mechanisms that enable injury expansion following aSAH are still not fully understood, and only a limited number of pharmacological treatments have been proven effective. Recent data suggest that neuroinflammation has a pivotal effect in injury expansion and neurological deficits [11–13]. Immune cells from the periphery are recruited into the brain parenchyma, and their activated forms release inflammatory cytokines [14,15]. Vessels affected by cerebral vasospasm have been found to have an elevated leukocyte adhesion capacity, resulting in delayed neurologic deterioration [16,17].

Numerous previous clinical trials have investigated the use of various anti-inflammatory drugs in aSAH patients to improve mortality and functional outcomes. In this meta-analysis, we aim to examine the available evidence and identify effective drug interventions that could improve functional outcomes and survival rates in aSAH patients.

2. Materials and Methods

To carry out this systematic review, we utilized the Cochrane Collaboration format [18] and adhered to the PRISMA checklist (see Supplementary Figure S1) [19]. The study was registered in the "*International Prospective Register of Systematic Reviews*" (PROSPERO) in 2023 (CRD42023395375), and a comprehensive, predetermined protocol can be obtained upon request.

2.1. Search Strategy for Identification of Studies

The authors performed a systematic search of the Pubmed database (http://www.ncbi.nlm.nih.gov/pubmed) using the terms "aneurysmal subarachnoid hemorrhage", "SAH", and "subarachnoid hemorrhage". The search was limited to randomized controlled trials, human studies, and English-language articles. The authors screened the articles for randomized placebo, controlled trials investigating anti-inflammatory drug therapies. The literature search encompassed all results until 31 March 2023. The inclusion criteria were developed based on the PICOS (population, intervention, comparator, outcomes, and study design) framework [20]. The following criteria were applied: patients suffered from aSAH; anti-inflammatory drug therapies were implemented; results were compared to a placebo arm; all results of the prespecified endpoints were reported; and the trials were defined as prospective, randomized, placebo-controlled, and double-blinded. The authors excluded certain types of results, such as reviews, letters, study protocols, conference abstracts, unpublished manuscripts, animal experiments, and studies with insufficient data (e.g., randomized controlled trials without a placebo arm). Furthermore, we conducted a search for studies that matched our inclusion and exclusion criteria in previous meta-analyses and systematic reviews. The identified articles underwent a stepwise evaluation process: Initial screening of study titles, followed by assessment of corresponding abstracts, and in case of uncertainty, the full-text screening by two authors (JW and EG) until all retrieved studies were either included or excluded.

2.2. Types of Studies

Randomized, double-blind, placebo-controlled clinical trials that evaluated the efficacy of anti-inflammatory treatment in improving the outcome and survival rates of aneurysmal subarachnoid hemorrhage were included. Trials without survival or neurological outcome data were excluded. Trials that specifically investigated elderly or geriatric aSAH patients (>60 years) were excluded. Neurological outcome was measured using the modified Rankin Scale (mRS). If an article presented numerical data for individual mRS classes, the data were documented based on the definition of a poor outcome as a score ranging from 3 to 6 on the mRS scale, while a score ≤ 2 was considered indicative of a good outcome [21]. If a study presented the percentage of patients with a defined outcome event, the absolute numbers were computed using the provided percentages.

2.3. Data Extraction and Quality Evaluation

Baseline data extracted from the studies included the study names, first authors, publication year, country, number of centers (whether mono-, bi-, or multicentric), key trial design characteristics (such as randomization method, allocation method, presence of missing data, lack of reported outcome, and utilization of intention-to-treat analysis), as well as other pertinent information.

2.4. Statistics

The meta-analyses were performed using Review Manger Web (RevMan Web Version 5.4.1 from The Cochrane Collaboration). Statistical heterogeneity was assessed using the χ^2, while inconsistency was evaluated using the I^2 statistics. Substantial heterogeneity was considered when the I^2 value reached 50% or higher. The weight of each individual trial's contribution to the treatment effect estimation was determined based on the study sample size. Data from a multi-arm trial that involved different dosage regimens were combined to create a unified group for inclusion in the pairwise meta-analysis [22]. To assess publication bias for the defined endpoints of survival and neurological outcome, three methods were applied. Firstly, funnel plots were generated to visually examine the publication bias of the included trials. Secondly, an Egger regression analysis was conducted to statistically evaluate the symmetry of the funnel plot. The likelihood of publication bias was determined using the two-tailed Egger regression intercept test, with a significance threshold set at 5% [23]. Thirdly, Begg's test was utilized to evaluate the symmetry of the data [24]. MedCalc (Version 20.123 for Windows) was used to perform both Egger's and Begg's tests. Pooled odds ratio (OR) estimates, using a random effects model, were used to express the effect sizes. Analyses were conducted for both death and poor outcome.

3. Results

3.1. Literature Search

Based on the search strategy, a total of 967 English articles (Figure 1) were deemed eligible. Following the evaluation of the titles, abstracts, and full texts, 953 articles were excluded. Ultimately, 14 articles encompassing 1759 patients were included for the meta-analysis.

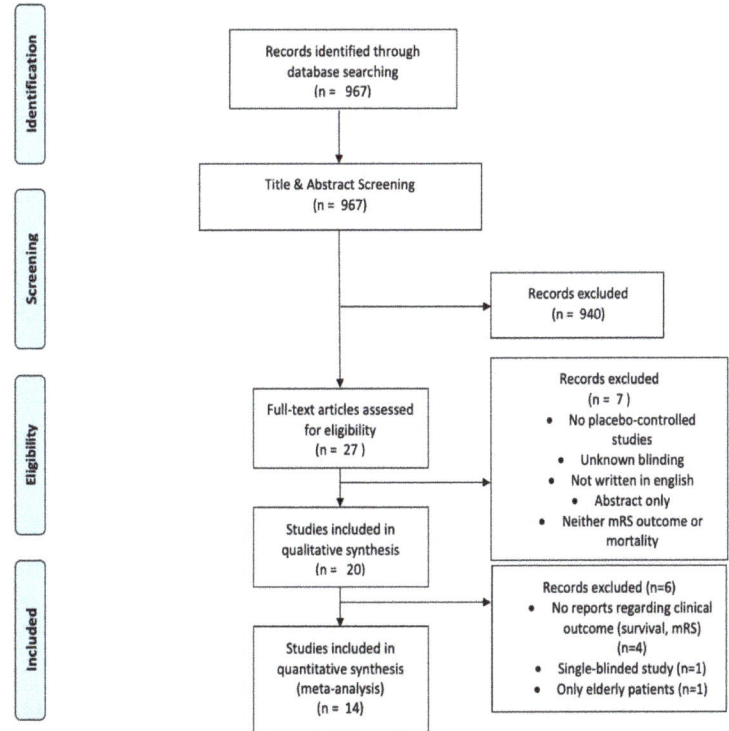

Figure 1. PRISMA flow chart showing the study selection of the present meta-analysis.

3.2. Characteristics of Included Studies

The included studies were published from 1989 to 2022. Table 1 shows the major characteristics of the anti-inflammatory drug interventions of the 14 included trials [25–38]. The participants included in each study were all aneurysmal SAH patients. The duration of treatments varied from 24 h to 21 days. One prospective, double-blind, and placebo-controlled trial was designed as a multi-arm trial [34]. Data were included by combining groups into the pairwise meta-analysis of our dichotomous endpoints. Further identified anti-inflammatory prospective studies in aSAH that did not fulfill our inclusion criteria due to single-blinded design, unknown blinding method, investigating elderly patients only, written in other languages than English, unavailable data for the primary endpoints of this meta-analysis, or the lack of placebo arms are provided in the Supplementary Table S1 [39–51].

Table 1. Major characteristics of anti-inflammatory studies included in the present meta-analysis.

Name	Year	Treatments and Sample Size	Doses	Treatment Duration	Recruiting Area
Chou et al. [25]	2008	Simvastatin = 19 versus SNT = 20	80 mg oral daily	Until discharge from NICU or until 21 days	United States of America
Diringer et al. [26]	2016	Simvastatin = 12 versus SNT = 12	80 mg oral daily	21 days	United States of America
Garcia-Pastor et al. [27]	2022	Dapsone = 26 versus SNT = 22	100 mg oral daily	Within 5 days after ictus until day 15	Mexico
Garg et al. [28]	2013	Simvastatin = 19 versus SNT = 19	80 mg daily for 14 days	14 days	India
Gomis et al. [29]	2010	Methylprednisolone = 49 versus SNT = 46	16 mg/kg intravenous daily	3 days	France
Hop et al. [30]	2000	ASA = 24 versus SNT = 26	100 mg suppositories daily	21 days	Netherlands
Katayama et al. [31]	2007	Hydrocortisone = 35 versus SNT = 36	1200 mg/d (day 0–10), 600 mg/d (day 11–12), 300 mg/d (day 13–14) intravenously	14 days	Japan
Kirkpatrick et al. [32]	2014	Simvastatin = 391 versus SNT = 412	40 mg oral daily	3 weeks	UK, Canada, Colombia, Italy, Russia, Singapore, Sweden, Uruguay, USA
Martini et al. [33]	2022	Epoxide hydrolase inhibitor = 10 versus SNT = 10	10 mg oral daily	10 days	United States of America
Suzuki et al. [34]	1989	OKY-046 = 172 versus SNT = 86	80 mg/day (low-dose group) 400 mg/day (high-dose group) intravenously	10 to 14 days	Japan
Tseng et al. [35]	2005	Pravastatin = 40 versus SNT = 40	40 mg oral daily	Within 3 days after ictus for 14 days or until discharge	United Kingdom
Van den Bergh et al. [36]	2006	ASA = 83 versus SNT = 70	100 mg suppositories daily	14 days	Netherlands
Vergouwen et al. [37]	2009	Simvastatin = 14 versus SNT = 16	80 mg oral daily	Within 3 days after SAH until day 14	Netherlands
Woo et al. [38]	2020	Cerebrolysin = 25 versus SNT = 25	30 mL daily for 14 days	14 days	Hong Kong

3.3. Risk of Bias and Quality Assessment

All included trials used a double-blinded design to minimize performance bias and detection bias of the personnel and patients. Furthermore, all trials were defined as randomized trials. The randomization technique was not reported in seven trials [25–27,29–31,34]. All prespecified endpoints are reported with the corresponding outcomes. Generally, no prospective, randomized, double-blind, and placebo-controlled trial showed characteristics that might indicate a high risk of bias. The frequency of the individual bias of each trial and the overall bias assessment are displayed in Figure 2. The detailed quality assessment protocol regarding risk of bias and author judgments for the individual studies are given in Supplementary Table S2.

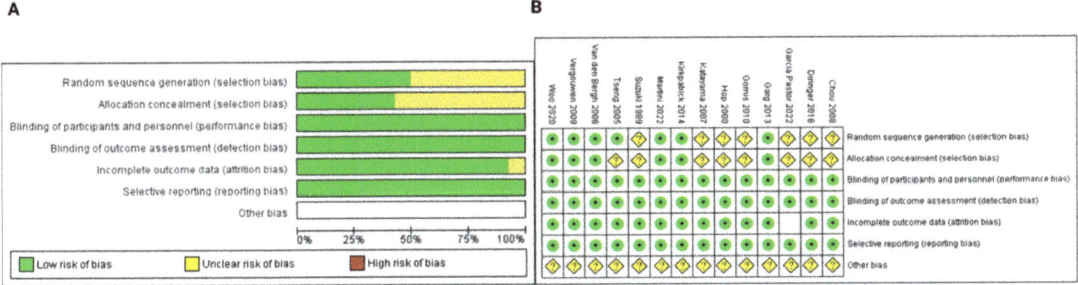

Figure 2. (**A**) Risk of bias evaluation for each kind of bias. (**B**) Summary of risk of bias of the individual randomized controlled trials (reviewers' judgments about each risk of bias characteristic of the included studies: "+" constitutes low risk; "?" constitutes unclear risk).

3.4. Impact of Anti-Inflammatory Therapy in Aneurysmal SAH on Survival

A total of 13 studies met our selection criteria and reported data regarding survival [25–30,32–38]. A total of 1689 patients were randomized into either anti-inflammatory (n = 885) or placebo treatment (n = 804). A total of 78 patients (8.8%) out of 885 in the anti-inflammatory treatment arm died, and 85 (10.6%) of the 804 patients in the control arms died. The outcome evaluation ranged from one month to one year after treatment. The overall odds ratio (Figure 3) for death in the pooled analysis was 0.81 (95% CI: 0.55–1.19) (p = 0.28). No significant heterogeneity was present (I^2 = 8%, p = 0.36). No studies were identified that indicated a significant positive or negative impact of anti-inflammatory therapy on the outcome endpoint of "death".

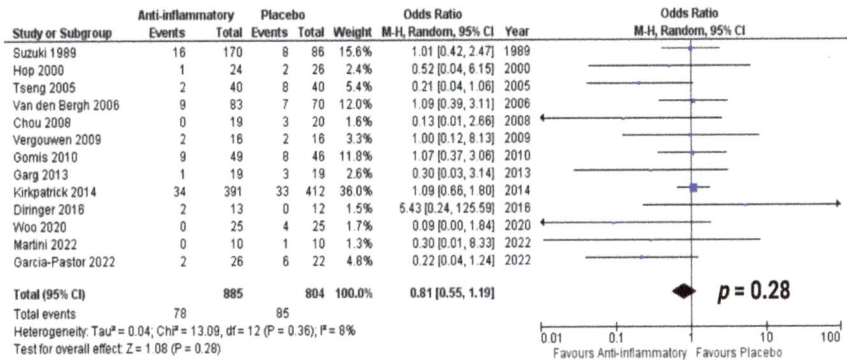

Figure 3. Forest Plots displaying OR and 95% CI estimates for death in studies evaluating anti-inflammatory therapies compared to conventional therapy in aSAH [25–30,32–38]. Squares constitute the odds ratio; the bigger the square, the greater the weight given because of the narrower 95% CI. Diamond shows the odds ratio of the overall data.

3.5. Impact of Anti-Inflammatory Therapy in Aneurysmal SAH on Neurological Outcome

A total of 9 studies met our selection criteria and reported data regarding neurological outcome, which enabled a dichotomization into mRS $\leq$ 2 or mRS > 2 [25–27,29–32,35,38]. A total of 1223 patients were randomized into either anti-inflammatory (n = 601) or control treatment (n = 622). In total, 428 patients (71.2%) out of 601 in the anti-inflammatory treatment arm achieved a good neurological outcome (mRS $\leq$ 2), and 419 (67.4%) of the 622 patients in the placebo arms achieved a favorable outcome. The outcome evaluation ranged from one month to one year after treatment. The overall odds ratio (Figure 4) for mRS $\leq$ 2 in the pooled analysis was 1.48 (95% CI: 0.95–2.32) (p = 0.08). No significant heterogeneity was present (I^2 = 45%, p = 0.07). One study investigating the effect of dapsone reported a beneficial effect regarding functional outcome as endpoint [27]. Furthermore, cerebrolysin also resulted in an increased probability to achieve a favorable outcome compared to placebo treatment [38].

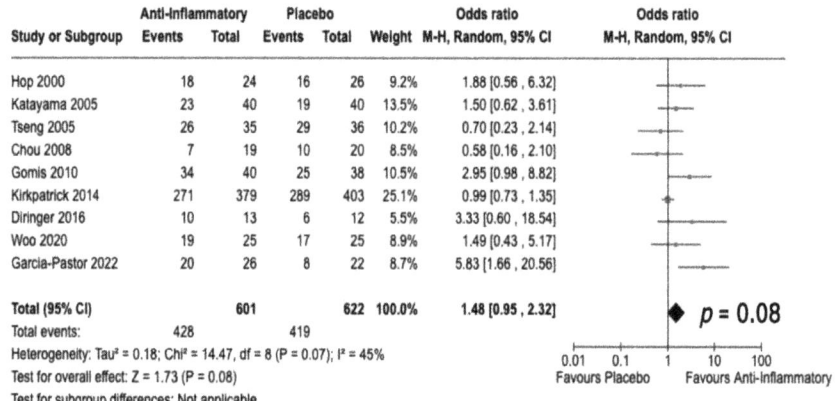

Figure 4. Forest Plots displaying OR and 95% CI estimates for a good neurological outcome (using mRS grading: mRS $\leq$ 2) in studies evaluating anti-inflammatory therapies compared to placebo therapy in aneurysmal SAH [25–27,29–32,35,38]. Squares constitute the odds ratio; the bigger the square, the greater the weight given because of the narrower 95% CI. Diamond shows the odds ratio of the overall data.

3.6. Publication Bias

In order to ensure a reliable assessment, several measures were implemented to examine the presence of publication bias. Firstly, a comprehensive literature search strategy was applied. Secondly, the selected studies included in this meta-analysis strictly adhered to the predefined inclusion and exclusion criteria. Thirdly, publication bias was evaluated using funnel plots (see Figure 5) for the endpoints (survival and favorable mRS outcome ($\leq$2)). Finally, statistical analyses of publication bias using Egger´s and Begg´s tests were performed. The data points for survival analysis were all positioned within the inverted funnel, indicating no visually apparent significant publication bias in relation to the survival analysis.

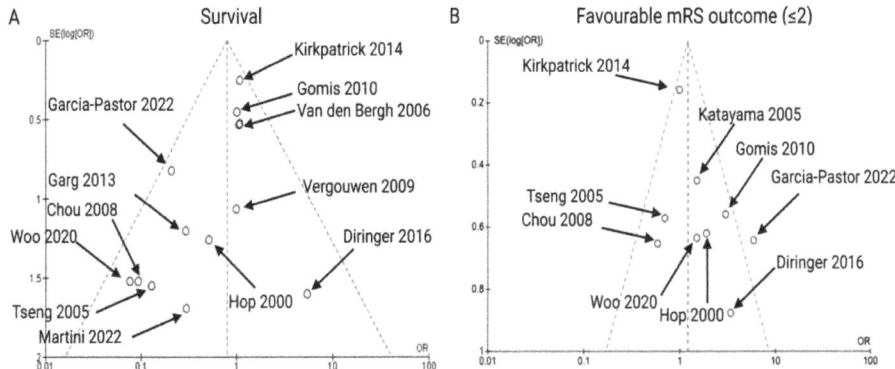

Figure 5. (**A**) Funnel plot visualizing the analysis of publications bias for the endpoint survival in 13 studies [25–30,32–38]. (**B**) Funnel plot visualizing the analysis of publications bias for the endpoint neurological outcome in nine studies [25–27,29–32,35,38].

Following the visual examination for publication bias, both Egger´s and Begg´s tests were conducted to investigate the presence of publication bias for the primary outcomes. Regarding mortality, Egger´s test indicated a statistically significant publication bias ($p = 0.03$, intercept $= -1.05$, 95% CI -1.99–-0.11), while Begg´s test revealed a Kendall's tau of -0.23 ($p = 0.27$). We identified one study investigating dapsone in aSAH with a very high effect size in the bottom-right corner of the funnel plot regarding favorable mRS outcome analysis [26]. Hence, there might be the risk that there is an underbelly of unpublished studies with similar standard errors, but small and non-significant effects. Furthermore, Egger´s test did not indicate any significant publication bias concerning the endpoint of "favourable mRS outcome (≤ 2)" ($p = 0.10$, intercept $= 1.23$, 95% CI -0.30–2.76), and Begg's test yielded a Kendall's tau of 0.29 ($p = 0.25$).

4. Discussion

The present meta-analysis summarized available data on anti-inflammatory therapy in aSAH and suggests a potential need for further trials investigating anti-inflammatory therapies using dapsone or corticosteroids. These drugs may positively influence the neurological outcome after aSAH. Our results indicate that anti-inflammatory therapy may have a positive effect on functional outcome. This provides valuable evidence for clinicians when considering the prescription of effective medications for patients with aSAH. Nimodipine remains the benchmark medical drug therapy for preventing DCI and influencing the outcome in aSAH patients [3,52]. In the following section, we will discuss the findings of the present meta-analysis and debate the classes of investigated anti-inflammatory drugs.

4.1. COX Inhibition

Cyclooxygenase (COX) is a bifunctional enzyme that acts as a cyclo-oxygenase and catalase. The conversion of arachidonic acid to prostaglandins is facilitated by the enzymes COX-1 and COX-2. COX-1 synthesizes thromboxane A2, which induces platelet aggregation, vasoconstriction, and proliferation of smooth muscles. In contrast, COX-2 synthesizes prostacyclin, which induces vasodilation and relaxation of smooth muscles and antagonizes thromboxane A2 in the macrovascular endothelium [53,54]. Animal investigations have shown that arterial endothelial cells have an increased expression of COX-2 after SAH, while the expression of COX-1 remains unchanged [55]. Animal trials have shown that inhibiting COX-2 may prevent brain edema and preserve neurological functioning [56]. However, non-selective COX-2 inhibition by nonsteroidal anti-inflammatory medications, such as acetylsalicylic acid, might elevate the risk of re-bleeding, despite attenuating neuroinflammation in aSAH [57,58]. Although acetylsalicylic acid failed to significantly reduce the risk of a delayed ischemic neurological deficit and improve the functional outcome in prospective, double-blind, and placebo-controlled trials [30,36], there was a tendency to prescribe it, as its relative risk reduction for poor outcome was 21% [36]. Celecoxib, a selective COX-2 inhibitor, has not been prospectively investigated in randomized and double-blinded aSAH trials yet. A small clinical trial on subjects with intracerebral hemorrhage showed that celecoxib reduced hematoma and edema volume through its anti-inflammatory effect [59]. However, the current limited evidence for celecoxib therapy in aSAH is due to the failure of acetylsalicylic acid and the known increased risk of myocardial infarction with celecoxib therapy [60].

4.2. Thromboxane A2 Synthetase Inhibition

Thromboxane A2 (TXA_2) is a prothrombotic prostanoid that is predominantly synthesized via COX-1, COX-2, and TXA_2 synthase [61]. Furthermore, it is released by activated platelets in the case of inflammation or tissue injury [62]. Afterwards, TXA_2 binds to the TXA_2 receptor, resulting in smooth muscle cell constriction and platelet aggregation. Experimental SAH rat models showed that the SAH-induced regional blood flow reduction is closely linked to an increased expression of TXA_2 receptors in the smooth muscle cells of cerebral arteries and microvessels [63]. An increase of TXA_2 levels induces leukocyte aggregation and systemic inflammation. However, the already debated acetylsalicylic acid can reduce the TXA_2 levels by inactivating COX-1 [64], whereas nimodipine exerts no effect on serum thromboxane levels [65]. The prospective randomized double-blind trial of Suzuki et al. [34] showed a potential use of a thromboxane synthetase inhibitor in preventing vasospasm and infarcts in severe aSAH cases with Hunt & Hess grades III and IV. However, the results of this trial regarding functional outcome could not be included in the statistical analysis because they were not transferrable to the mRS scale.

4.3. Epoxide Hydrolase Inhibition

Soluble epoxide hydrolase is the metabolizing enzyme of epoxyeicosatrienoic acids, which oppose the expression of vascular cell adhesion molecule-1 (VCAM-1) by blocking the NF-κB translocation. The translocation NF-κB is an important part of the expression of the pro-inflammatory adhesion molecule VCAM-1 [66,67]. The consequence of this vascular inflammatory pathway is the development of a vasogenic edema, causing the extravasation of ions and proteins through a disturbed blood–brain barrier [68]. Animal experiments have shown that the genetic deletion or inhibition of soluble epoxide hydrolase results in a reduced expression of VCAM-1 in the cerebrovasculature, thereby attenuating the transmigration of infiltrating inflammatory cells [69,70]. Increased levels of VCAM-1 have been observed in the plasma or CSF of aSAH patients, and this inflammatory response is suggested to be an important part of vasogenic edema development [69,71]. The first human prospective, randomized, and placebo-controlled trial investigating soluble epoxide hydrolase inhibition was recently conducted by Martini et al. [33], which showed that the application is safe for humans, and there was no drug-associated mortality. Furthermore, it was revealed that soluble epoxide hydrolase inhibition resulted in increased serum levels of epoxyeicosatrienoic acids, whereas the cerebrospinal fluid levels of epoxyeicosatrienoic acids were not sufficiently increased by the application of the soluble epoxide hydrolase inhibitor. To date, the current evidence is limited by the low power size, and the results of the present meta-analysis cannot recommend a routine clinical application. Further larger trials of soluble epoxide hydrolase inhibitors with an improved CNS penetration might also provide information regarding the functional outcome.

4.4. Statins

Statins, which are commonly referred to as HMG-CoA reductase inhibitors, have pleiotropic effects, including anti-inflammatory actions and the attenuation of vasospasm. Statins enhance the expression and activity of endothelial nitric oxide synthase and reduce nitric oxide scavenging by free radicals [72,73]. Moreover, they can inhibit the activation and migration of inflammatory perivascular granulocytes [74,75], potentially attenuating or preventing cerebral vasospasms after aSAH. To date, eight randomized [25,26,28,35,37,44–46] and four large multicenter, prospective, randomized trials [32,43,49,51] have evaluated the use of simvastatin, atorvastatin, pitavastatin, or pravastatin in aSAH patients. However, 2 studies had a special focus on either elderly patients over 60 years [39] or a dose comparison of simvastatin without a placebo group [51]. The primary endpoints of these studies were the frequency of vasospasm, presence of DCI, and the functional outcome. A previous meta-analysis, which summarized the results of some of the aforementioned trials focused on the potential reduction of vasospasm (defined by transcranial doppler sonography), found no significant effect [76]. However, another meta-analysis, which exclusively focused on statins and the treatment duration, found that a statin therapy for 2 weeks may improve neurological outcome. Surprisingly, prolonged use for 3 weeks had no significant effect on neurological outcome [77]. In the present meta-analysis, we also could not observe a significant effect on mortality or functional outcome. Current evidence and guidelines do not recommend routine use of statins in aSAH [3,77,78]. To assess the impact of statin treatment over a duration of two weeks, it is necessary to conduct future large-scale trials. The recently published AHA/ASA 2023 aSAH guideline does not recommend the routine use of statin therapy regarding the prevention of delayed cerebral ischemia [4].

4.5. Cerebrolysin

Cerebrolysin is a low-molecular-weight neuropeptide compound with free amino acids that is derived from the porcine brain tissue. Animal experiments have shown that cerbrolysin has anti-inflammatory properties that can be beneficial in cerebral ischemic stroke. By inducing the expression of anti-inflammatory factors and promoting microglia polarization towards an anti-inflammatory type, cerebrolysin was found to reduce the ischemic infarct volume [79]. Randomized placebo-controlled clinical studies investigating the effect of cerebrolysin in acute ischemic stroke have shown improved 3-month functional outcomes regarding the mRS [80–85]. A 10-year retrospective investigation of cerebrolysin treatment in severe aSAH patients found an increase in the survival rates at the 3-month mark for individuals who underwent surgical intervention for aSAH [86]. Woo et al. [38] provided the first results on cerebrolysin in aSAH patients from a prospective randomized double-blind trial. Cerebrolysin appeared to be a safe drug, and mortality was reduced in the cerebrolysin group compared to the placebo group. However, the study size did not allow for this conclusion, and the results regarding functional outcome were also neutral. However, future trials will need to explore cerebrolysin in a larger cohort and with an earlier intervention time-window because significant improvements in 3-month outcomes were found in trials investigating cerebrolysin in ischemic stroke when it was administered within 6 h after hospital admission [82,86].

4.6. Dapsone

Dapsone, also known as 4,4′-diamino-diphenylsulfone, is a neuroprotective compound that acts by suppressing glutamate-mediated excitotoxicity and possesses anti-inflammatory properties [87,88]. The anti-inflammatory properties of dapsone are attributed to its ability to hinder the calcium-dependent actions of neutrophils, which includes the suppression of harmful oxidants and proteases released by these cells, leading to tissue damage. Furthermore, dapsone irreversibly inhibits myeloperoxidase, blocks peroxidase functioning in eosinophils, inhibits the synthesis of products by 5-lipoxygenase products, and decreases the levels of neurotoxic free radicals [87–90]. A prospective randomized and double-blind trial investigating dapsone in acute ischemic stroke revealed that patients receiving dapsone had significant improved neurological functioning at 2 months after acute ischemic stroke compared to the placebo group [90]. To date, only one trial has analyzed the use of dapsone in aSAH patients [27]. Our meta-analysis revealed that this study showed the most promising effect in terms of the probability of a favorable outcome, as defined by the mRS. This beneficial effect appears to be mainly due to the protective role of dapsone in reducing the incidence of vasospasms and DCI. In the placebo group, DCI was present in 63.6% of the patients, while only 26.9% of the patients in the dapsone group had DCI [27]. Future multicenter trials will be necessary to confirm these findings and could also focus on physiological investigations of cerebral blood flow.

4.7. Corticosteroids

Corticosteroids are frequently used anti-inflammatory drugs in neurosurgical pathologies due to their diverse functioning as mineralocorticoid or anti-inflammatory drugs. However, there is currently no evidence or guideline supporting the use of corticosteroids to improve neurological outcomes after aSAH [91]. Guidelines suggest maintaining euvolemia in patients with symptomatic delayed cerebral ischemia to reduce the progression and severity of delayed cerebral ischemia, supported by class I evidence [3,4,92–94]. Early administration of fludrocortisone was shown to decrease natriuretic diuresis, maintain euvolemia, and reduce symptomatic vasospasm in a study by Nakagawa et al. [95]. Vasospasm is associated with the inflammatory response after aSAH [96], as shown by prospectively recorded serum interleukin-6 levels in 80 patients that were associated with higher Hunt & Hess grades, development of seizure, cerebral vasospasms, and chronic hydrocephalus [97]. Therefore, corticosteroid therapy is assumed to decrease vasospasm by attenuating the inflammatory response. Four investigations analyzed the impact of corticosteroids with minimal mineralocorticoid functions: two trials analyzed methylprednisolone [29,98], whereas two trials utilized dexamethasone [99,100]. Although one randomized controlled trial by Gomis et al. [29] showed a significant reduction of symptomatic vasospasm in high-grade aSAH patients, this effect did not result in a significant improvement of functional outcomes compared to the placebo group. However, the lower boundary of the 95% CI was 0.98 in our pooled analysis, suggesting at least a tendency towards the administration of corticosteroids. Schürkämper et al. [100] investigated dexamethasone in a retrospective study of 242 aSAH patients and found that high-dose (>12 mg/d or >5 days) dexamethasone treatment resulted in an increased probability of favorable outcome compared to those receiving a lower total dose (<12 mg/d or <5 days). However, these results are limited by the retrospective design, and the control group received low amounts of dexamethasone. The ongoing FINISHER trial (**F**ight **IN**flammation to **I**mprove Outcome after Aneurysmal **S**ubarachnoid **HE**mor**R**hage, Trial-Number: NCT05132920) will provide the first data from a prospective randomized placebo-controlled trial evaluating dexamethasone. The primary endpoint of this multicentric trial is the mRS at 6 months after aSAH [101]. This study may elucidate whether the potential benefit of corticosteroids is based on the anti-inflammatory functioning. Furthermore, our current knowledge is based on a combination of several inflammatory pathways that contribute to the inflammatory response after aSAH. Dexamethasone may be an option to simultaneously inhibit several pathways (see Supplementary Figure S2), as the inhibition of single pathways has not shown a significant effect thus far.

This meta-analysis suggests a potential benefit of dapsone or corticosteroids in the management of aSAH, but the conclusions are limited by the low quality of evidence. Furthermore, the present meta-analysis of anti-inflammatory drugs is also limited by the fact that those drugs have different targets and effects. Hence, it is difficult to convex generalizability from the results of each individual study. Nevertheless, even the recent AHA/ASA 2023 aSAH guideline also points out that the emerging data suggesting inflammation to contribute to brain injury in aSAH necessitates further study on glucocorticoid steroids because their safety and efficacy profile is not sufficiently investigated so far [4]. Future studies will have to focus on whether there are different subgroups of aSAH patients who might benefit from different anti-inflammatory drugs targeting individual pathways. Additionally, the findings of the present meta-analysis investigating anti-inflammatory drugs must be interpreted with caution due to different pharmacodynamics and pharmacological effects. Several of the included anti-inflammatory drugs have also other functions, which are paramount regarding the care for aSAH patients. For instance, COX-1 inhibitors have also fundamental effects regarding the inhibition of platelet aggregation, whereas corticosteroids also act on the hemostatic system by increasing clotting factor levels and platelet counts [102–104]. The present analysis includes small studies with low statistical power and significant findings, while there are no studies with low power and non-significant results for mortality. Therefore, there may be a publication bias. A major limitation of the evaluation of the neurological outcome are the heterogeneous timepoints of the endpoints of the included studies and the different grades of clinical severity of aSAH, which confound our results. Ultimately, more rigorous data from large, prospective, randomized controlled trials are needed to evaluate the efficacy of dapsone or dexamethasone in the management of aSAH.

5. Conclusions

There was no difference in mortality between conventional therapy and anti-inflammatory therapy in patients with aneurysmal subarachnoid hemorrhage. However, certain individual anti-inflammatory therapies, such as dapsone and corticosteroids, may have a positive impact on functional outcomes. To establish sufficient evidence regarding the efficacy of anti-inflammatory therapy in aSAH, further multicenter, randomized, double-blind, and placebo-controlled trials are needed.

Supplementary Materials: The following supporting information can be downloaded at: https://www.mdpi.com/article/10.3390/jcm12124165/s1, Table S1: Characteristics of excluded anti-inflammatory studies; Table S2: Quality assessment of prospective randomized double-blind, and placebo-controlled trials; Figure S1: PRISMA checklist summarizing the checklist items and the location of the items in the present meta-analysis [105], Figure S2: Illustrative summary of the potential anti-inflammatory functioning and avenues influenced by corticosteroid therapy in aneurysmal subarachnoid hemorrhage.

Author Contributions: Conceptualization, E.G. and J.W.; methodology, E.G. and J.W.; data curation, E.G. and J.W.; writing—original draft preparation, E.G. and J.W.; writing—review and editing, A.G., M.V., M.V. and E.G.; visualization, E.G. and J.W.; supervision, E.G. All authors have read and agreed to the published version of the manuscript.

Funding: This research received no external funding.

Institutional Review Board Statement: This study was conducted according to the guidelines of the Declaration of Helsinki and no approval was necessary in case of a meta-analysis.

Informed Consent Statement: Written informed consent was not needed due to the retrospective design. The local ethics committee waived patient informed consent for this retrospective observational study.

Data Availability Statement: All data are included in this manuscript.

Acknowledgments: The graphical abstract was created using BioRender. The authors thank Jenny Messall for providing assistance in the design of Supplementary Figure S2. The present publication was funded by the Open Access Publishing Fund of Leipzig University supported by the German Research Foundation within the program Open Access Publation Funding.

Conflicts of Interest: The authors declare no conflict of interest.

References

1. Neifert, S.N.; Chapman, E.K.; Martini, M.L.; Shuman, W.H.; Schupper, A.J.; Oermann, E.K.; Mocco, J.; Macdonald, R.L. Aneurysmal Subarachnoid Hemorrhage: The Last Decade. *Transl. Stroke Res.* **2020**, *12*, 428–446. [CrossRef]
2. Etminan, N.; Chang, H.S.; Hackenberg, K.; de Rooij, N.K.; Vergouwen, M.D.I.; Rinkel, G.J.E.; Algra, A. Worldwide Incidence of Aneurysmal Subarachnoid Hemorrhage According to Region, Time Period, Blood Pressure, and Smoking Prevalence in the Population: A Systematic Review and Meta-analysis. *JAMA Neurol.* **2019**, *76*, 588–597. [CrossRef]
3. Connolly, E.S., Jr.; Rabinstein, A.A.; Carhuapoma, J.R.; Derdeyn, C.P.; Dion, J.; Higashida, R.T.; Hoh, B.L.; Kirkness, C.J.; Naidech, A.M.; Ogilvy, C.S.; et al. Guidelines for the management of aneurysmal subarachnoid hemorrhage: A guideline for healthcare professionals from the American Heart Association/american Stroke Association. *Stroke* **2012**, *43*, 1711–1737. [CrossRef]

4. Hoh, B.L.; Ko, N.U.; Amin-Hanjani, S.; Chou, S.H.-Y.; Cruz-Flores, S.; Dangayach, N.S.; Derdeyn, C.P.; Du, R.; Hänggi, D.; Hetts, S.W.; et al. 2023 Guideline for the Management of Patients with Aneurysmal Subarachnoid Hemorrhage: A Guideline From the American Heart Association/American Stroke Association. *Stroke* **2023**. [CrossRef]
5. Tjahjadi, M.; Heinen, C.; König, R.; Rickels, E.; Wirtz, C.R.; Woischneck, D.; Kapapa, T. Health-Related Quality of Life after Spontaneous Subarachnoid Hemorrhage Measured in a Recent Patient Population. *World Neurosurg.* **2013**, *79*, 296–307. [CrossRef] [PubMed]
6. Taufique, Z.; May, T.; Meyers, E.; Falo, C.; Mayer, S.A.; Agarwal, S.; Park, S.; Connolly, E.S.; Claassen, J.; Schmidt, J.M. Predictors of Poor Quality of Life 1 Year after Subarachnoid Hemorrhage. *Neurosurgery* **2016**, *78*, 256–264. [CrossRef]
7. Al-Khindi, T.; Macdonald, R.L.; Schweizer, T.A. Cognitive and Functional Outcome after Aneurysmal Subarachnoid Hemorrhage. *Stroke* **2010**, *41*, e519–e536. [CrossRef] [PubMed]
8. Eagles, M.E.; Tso, M.K.; Macdonald, R.L. Cognitive impairment, functional outcome, and delayed cerebral ischemia after aneurysmal subarachnoid hemorrhage. *World Neurosurg.* **2019**, *124*, e558–e562. [CrossRef]
9. Roos, Y.B.; de Haan, R.J.; Beenen, L.F.; Groen, R.J.; Albrecht, K.W.; Vermeulen, M. Complications and outcome in patients with aneurysmal subarachnoid haemorrhage: A prospective hospital based cohort study in the Netherlands. *J. Neurol. Neurosurg. Psychiatry* **2000**, *68*, 337–341. [CrossRef]
10. Platz, J.; Güresir, E.; Vatter, H.; Berkefeld, J.; Seifert, V.; Raabe, A.; Beck, J. Unsecured intracranial aneurysms and induced hypertension safe? *Neurocrit. Care* **2011**, *14*, 168–175. [CrossRef] [PubMed]
11. Caffes, N.; Kurland, D.B.; Gerzanich, V.; Simard, J.M. Glibenclamide for the treatment of ischemic and hemorrhagic stroke. *Int. J. Mol. Sci.* **2015**, *16*, 4973–4984. [CrossRef]
12. Makino, H.; Tada, Y.; Wada, K.; Liang, E.I.; Chang, M.; Mobashery, S.; Kanematsu, Y.; Kurihara, C.; Palova, E.; Kanematsu, M.; et al. Pharmacological stabilization of intracranial aneurysms in mice: A feasibility study. *Stroke* **2012**, *43*, 2450–2456. [CrossRef]
13. Güresir, E.; Gräff, I.; Seidel, M.; Bauer, H.; Coch, C.; Diepenseifen, C.; Dohmen, C.; Engels, S.; Hadjiathanasiou, A.; Heister, U.; et al. Aneurysmal Subarachnoid Hemorrhage during the Shutdown for COVID-19. *J. Clin. Med.* **2022**, *11*, 2555. [CrossRef]
14. Moraes, L.; Grille, S.; Morelli, P.; Mila, R.; Trias, N.; Brugnini, A.; Lluberas, N.; Biestro, A.; Lens, D. Immune cells subpopulations in cerebrospinal fluid and peripheral blood of patients with Aneurysmal Subarachnoid Hemorrhage. *Springerplus* **2015**, *4*, 195. [CrossRef]
15. Kooijman, E.; Nijboer, C.H.; van Velthoven, C.T.; Kavelaars, A.; Kesecioglu, J.; Heijnen, C.J. The rodent endovascular puncture model of subarachnoid hemorrhage: Mechanisms of brain damage and therapeutic strategies. *J. Neuroinflamm.* **2014**, *11*, 2. [CrossRef]
16. Provencio, J.J.; Badjatia, N. Participants in the International Multi-disciplinary Consensus Conference on Multimodality Monitoring. Monitoring inflammation (including fever) in acute brain injury. *Neurocrit. Care* **2014**, *21* (Suppl. 2), S177–S186. [CrossRef]
17. Xu, H.-L.; Garcia, M.; Testai, F.; Vetri, F.; Barabanova, A.; Pelligrino, D.A.; Paisansathan, C. Pharmacologic blockade of vascular adhesion protein-1 lessens neurologic dysfunction in rats subjected to subarachnoid hemorrhage. *Brain Res.* **2014**, *1586*, 83–89. [CrossRef] [PubMed]
18. Higgins, J.; Green, S. *Cochrane Handbook for Systematic Reviews of Interventions Version 5.1.0.*; Cochrane Collab: London, UK, 2011; Available online: www.cochrane-handbook.org (accessed on 1 September 2022).
19. Liberati, M.; Tetzlaff, J.; Altman, D.G.; PRISMA Group. Preferred reporting items for systematic reviews and meta-analyses: The PRISMA statement. *PLoS Med.* **2009**, *6*, e1000097. [CrossRef] [PubMed]
20. Schardt, C.; Adams, M.B.; Owens, T.; Keitz, S.; Fontelo, P. Utilization of the PICO framework to improve searching PubMed for clinical questions. *BMC Med. Inform. Decis. Mak.* **2007**, *7*, 16. [CrossRef]
21. Lampmann, T.; Hadjiathanasiou, A.; Asoglu, H.; Wach, J.; Kern, T.; Vatter, H.; Güresir, E. Early Serum Creatinine Levels after Aneurysmal Subarachnoid Hemorrhage Predict Functional Neurological Outcome after 6 Months. *J. Clin. Med.* **2022**, *11*, 4753. [CrossRef] [PubMed]
22. Rücker, G.; Cates, C.J.; Schwarzer, G. Methods for including information from multi-arm trials in pairwise meta-analysis. *Res. Synth. Methods* **2017**, *8*, 392–403. [CrossRef]
23. Egger, M.; Smith, G.D.; Schneider, M.; Minder, C. Bias in meta-analysis detected by a simple, graphical test. *BMJ* **1997**, *315*, 629–634. [CrossRef]
24. Begg, C.B.; Mazumdar, M. Operating Characteristics of a Rank Correlation Test for Publication Bias. *Biometrics* **1994**, *50*, 1088–1101. [CrossRef] [PubMed]
25. Chou, S.H.; Smith, E.E.; Badjatia, N.; Nogueira, R.G.; Sims, J.R., 2nd; Ogilvy, C.S.; Rordorf, G.A.; Ayata, C. A randomized, double-blind, placebo-controlled pilot study of simvastatin in aneurysmal subarachnoid hemorrhage. *Stroke* **2008**, *39*, 2891–2893. [CrossRef]
26. Diringer, M.N.; Dhar, R.; Scalfani, M.; Zazulia, A.R.; Chicoine, M.; Powers, W.J.; Derdeyn, C.P. Effect of High-Dose Simvastatin on Cerebral Blood Flow and Static Autoregulation in Subarachnoid Hemorrhage. *Neurocrit. Care* **2015**, *25*, 56–63. [CrossRef]
27. García-Pastor, C.; de Llano, J.P.N.-G.; Balcázar-Padrón, J.C.; Tristán-López, L.; Rios, C.; Díaz-Ruíz, A.; Rodríguez-Hernandez, L.A.; Nathal, E. Neuroprotective effect of dapsone in patients with aneurysmal subarachnoid hemorrhage: A prospective, randomized, double-blind, placebo-controlled clinical trial. *Neurosurg. Focus* **2022**, *52*, E12. [CrossRef]

28. Garg, K.; Sinha, S.; Kale, S.S.; Chandra, P.S.; Suri, A.; Singh, M.M.; Kumar, R.; Sharma, M.S.; Pandey, R.M.; Sharma, B.S.; et al. Role of simvastatin in prevention of vasospasm and improving functional outcome after aneurysmal subarachnoid hemorrhage: A prospective, randomized, double-blind, placebo-controlled pilot trial. *Br. J. Neurosurg.* **2013**, *27*, 181–186. [CrossRef]
29. Gomis, P.; Graftieaux, J.P.; Sercombe, R.; Hettler, D.; Scherpereel, B.; Rousseaux, P. Randomized, double-blind, placebo-controlled, pilot trial of high-dose methylprednisolone in aneurysmal subarachnoid hemorrhage. *J. Neurosurg.* **2010**, *112*, 681–688. [CrossRef] [PubMed]
30. Hop, J.W.; Rinkel, G.J.E.; Algra, A.; van der Sprenkel, J.B.; van Gijn, J. Randomized pilot trial of postoperative aspirin in subarachnoid hemorrhage. *Neurology* **2000**, *54*, 872–878. [CrossRef] [PubMed]
31. Katayama, Y.; Haraoka, J.; Hirabayashi, H.; Kawamata, T.; Kawamoto, K.; Kitahara, T.; Kojima, J.; Kuroiwa, T.; Mori, T.; Moro, N.; et al. A randomized controlled trial of hydrocortisone against hyponatremia in patients with aneurysmal subarachnoid hemorrhage. *Stroke* **2007**, *38*, 2373–2375. [CrossRef] [PubMed]
32. Kirkpatrick, P.J.; Turner, C.L.; Smith, C.; Hutchinson, P.J.; Murray, G.D.; STASH Collaborators. Simvastatin in aneurysmal subarachnoid haemorrhage (STASH): A multicentre randomised phase 3 trial. *Lancet Neurol.* **2014**, *13*, 666–675. [CrossRef]
33. Martini, R.P.; Siler, D.; Cetas, J.; Alkayed, N.J.; Allen, E.; Treggiari, M.M. A Double-Blind, Randomized, Placebo-Controlled Trial of Soluble Epoxide Hydrolase Inhibition in Patients with Aneurysmal Subarachnoid Hemorrhage. *Neurocrit. Care* **2022**, *36*, 905–915. [CrossRef]
34. Suzuki, S.; Sano, K.; Handa, H.; Asano, T.; Tamura, A.; Yonekawa, Y.; Ono, H.; Tachibana, N.; Hanaoka, K. Clinical study of OKY-046, a thromboxane synthetase inhibitor, in prevention of cerebral vasospasms and delayed cerebral ischemic symptoms after subarachnoid haemorrhage due to aneurysmal rupture: A randomized double-blind study. *Neurol. Res.* **1989**, *11*, 79–88. [CrossRef] [PubMed]
35. Tseng, M.Y.; Czosnyka, M.; Richards, H.; Pickard, J.D.; Kirkpatrick, P.J. Faculty Opinions recommendation of Effects of acute treatment with pravastatin on cerebral vasospasm, autoregulation, and delayed ischemic deficits after aneurysmal subarachnoid hemorrhage: A phase II randomized placebo-controlled trial. *Stroke* **2015**, *36*, 1627–1632. [CrossRef]
36. Van den Bergh, W.M.; lgra, A.; Dorhout Mees, S.M.; van Kooten, F.; Dirven, C.M.; van Gijn, J.; Vermeulen, M.; Rinkel, G.J.; MASH Study Group. Randomized controlled trial of acetylsalicylic acid in aneurysmal subarachnoid hemorrhage: The MASH study. *Stroke* **2006**, *37*, 2326–2330. [CrossRef]
37. Vergouwen, M.D.I.; Meijers, J.C.M.; Geskus, R.B.; Coert, B.A.; Horn, J.; Stroes, E.S.G.; Van Der Poll, T.; Vermeulen, M.; Roos, Y.B.W.E.M. Biologic Effects of Simvastatin in Patients with Aneurysmal Subarachnoid Hemorrhage: A Double-Blind, Placebo-Controlled Randomized Trial. *J. Cereb. Blood Flow Metab.* **2009**, *29*, 1444–1453. [CrossRef] [PubMed]
38. Woo, P.Y.M.; Ho, J.W.K.; Ko, N.M.W.; Li, R.P.T.; Jian, L.; Chu, A.C.H.; Kwan, M.C.L.; Chan, Y.; Wong, A.K.S.; Wong, H.-T.; et al. Randomized, placebo-controlled, double-blind, pilot trial to investigate safety and efficacy of Cerebrolysin in patients with aneurysmal subarachnoid hemorrhage. *BMC Neurol.* **2020**, *20*, 401. [CrossRef]
39. Chen, J.; Li, M.; Zhu, X.; Chen, L.; Yang, S.; Zhang, C.; Wu, T.; Feng, X.; Wang, Y.; Chen, Q. Atorvastatin reduces cerebral vasospasm and infarction after aneurysmal subarachnoid hemorrhage in elderly Chinese adults. *Aging* **2020**, *12*, 2939–2951. [CrossRef]
40. Fei, L.; Golwa, F. Topical application of dexamethasone to prevent cerebral vasospasm after aneurysmal subarachnoid haemorrhage: A pilot study. *Clin. Drug Investig.* **2007**, *27*, 827–832. [CrossRef]
41. Galea, J.; Ogungbenro, K.; Hulme, S.; Patel, H.; Scarth, S.; Hoadley, M.; Illingworth, K.; McMahon, C.J.; Tzerakis, N.; King, A.; et al. Reduction of inflammation after administration of interleukin-1 receptor antagonist following aneurysmal subarachnoid hemorrhage: Results of the Subcutaneous Interleukin-1Ra in SAH (SCIL-SAH) study. *J. Neurosurg.* **2018**, *128*, 515–523. [CrossRef] [PubMed]
42. Hasan, D.; Lindsay, K.W.; Wijdicks, E.F.; Murray, G.D.; Brouwers, P.J.; Bakker, W.H.; van Gijn, J.; Vermeulen, M. Effect of fludrocortisone acetate in patients with subarachnoid hemorrhage. *Stroke* **1989**, *20*, 1156–1161. [CrossRef]
43. Hashi, K.; Takakura, K.; Sano, K.; Ohta, T.; Saito, I.; Okada, K. Intravenous hydrocortisone in large doses in the treatment of delayed ischemic neurological deficits following subarachnoid hemorrhage—Results of a multi-center controlled double-blind clinical study. *No Shinkei= Brain Nerve* **1988**, *40*, 373–382.
44. Jaschinski, U.; Scherer, K.; Lichtwarck, M.; Forst, H. Impact of treatment with pravastatin on delayed ischemic disease and mortality after aneurysmal subarachnoid hemorrhage. *Crit. Care* **2008**, *12*, P112. [CrossRef]
45. Lynch, J.R.; Wang, H.; McGirt, M.J.; Floyd, J.; Friedman, A.H.; Coon, A.L.; Blessing, R.; Alexander, M.J.; Graffagnino, C.; Warner, D.S.; et al. Simvastatin reduces vasospasm after aneurysmal subarachnoid hemorrhage: Results of a pilot randomized clinical trial. *Stroke* **2005**, *36*, 2024–2026. [CrossRef]
46. Macedo, S.; Bello, Y.; Silva, A.; Siqueira, C.; Siqueira, S.; Brito, L. Effects of simvastatin in prevention of vasospasm in nontraumatic subarachnoid hemorrhage: Preliminary data. *Crit. Care* **2009**, *13*, P103. [CrossRef]
47. Mori, T.; Katayama, Y.; Kawamata, T.; Hirayama, T.; Khan, M.I.; Dellinger, R.P.; Waguespack, S.G.; Shah, K.; Turgeon, R.D.; Gooderham, P.A.; et al. Improved efficiency of hypervolemic therapy with inhibition of natriuresis by fludrocortisone in patients with aneurysmal subarachnoid hemorrhage. *J. Neurosurg.* **1999**, *91*, 947–952. [CrossRef]
48. Moro, N.; Katayama, Y.; Kojima, J.; Mori, T.; Kawamata, T. Prophylactic management of excessive natriuresis with hydrocortisone for efficient hypervolemic theerapy after subarachnoid hemorrhage. *Stroke* **2003**, *34*, 2807–2811. [CrossRef]

49. Naraoka, M.; Matsuda, N.; Shimamura, N.; Asano, K.; Akasaka, K.; Takemura, A.; Hasegawa, S.; Ohkuma, H. Long-acting statin for aneurysmal subarachnoid hemorrhage: A randomized, double-blind, placebo-controlled trial. *J. Cereb. Blood Flow Metab.* **2017**, *38*, 1190–1198. [CrossRef] [PubMed]
50. Singh, N.; Hopkins, S.J.; Hulme, S.; Galea, J.P.; Hoadley, M.; Vail, A.; Hutchinson, P.J.; Grainger, S.; Rothwell, N.J.; King, A.T.; et al. The effect of intravenous interleukin-1 receptor antagonist on inflammatory mediators in cerebrospinal fluid after subarachnoid haemorrhage: A phase II randomised controlled trial. *J. Neuroinflamm.* **2014**, *11*, 1. [CrossRef] [PubMed]
51. Wong, G.K.; Chan, D.Y.; Siu, D.Y.; Zee, B.C.; Poon, W.S.; Chan, M.T.; Gin, T.; Leung, M.; HDS-SAH Investigators. High-dose simvastatin for aneurysmal subarachnoid hemorrhage: Multicenter randomized controlled double-blinded clinical trial. *Stroke* **2015**, *46*, 382–388. [CrossRef] [PubMed]
52. Pickard, J.D.; Murray, G.D.; Illingworth, R.; Shaw, M.D.; Teasdale, G.M.; Foy, P.M.; Humphrey, P.R.; Lang, D.A.; Nelson, R.; Richards, P. Effect of oral nimodipine on cerebral infarction and outcome after subarachnoid haemorrhage: British aneurysm nimodipine trial. *BMJ* **1989**, *298*, 636–642. [CrossRef]
53. Rouzer, C.A.; Marnett, L.J. Structural and Chemical Biology of the Interaction of Cyclooxygenase with Substrates and Non-Steroidal Anti-Inflammory Drugs. *Chem. Rev.* **2020**, *120*, 7592–7641. [CrossRef]
54. Wu, F.; Liu, Z.; Li, G.; Zhou, L.; Huang, K.; Wu, Z.; Zhan, R.; Shen, J. Inflammation and Oxidative Stress: Potential Targets for Improving Prognosis After Subarachnoid Hemorrhage. *Front. Cell. Neurosci.* **2021**, *15*, 739506. [CrossRef]
55. Dinh, Y.R.T.; Jomaa, A.; Callebert, J.; Reynier-Rebuffel, A.-M.; Tedgui, A.; Savarit, A.; Sercombe, R. Overexpression of Cyclooxygenase-2 in Rabbit Basilar Artery Endothelial Cells after Subarachnoid Hemorrhage. *Neurosurgery* **2001**, *48*, 626–635. [CrossRef] [PubMed]
56. Ayer, R.; Jadhav, V.; Sugawara, T.; Zhang, J.H. The Neuroprotective Effects of Cyclooxygenase-2 Inhibition in a Mouse Model of Aneurysmal Subarachnoid Hemorrhage. *Acta Neurochir. Suppl.* **2011**, *111*, 145–149. [CrossRef]
57. Roumie, C.L.; Mitchel, E.F., Jr.; Kaltenbach, L.; Arbogast, P.G.; Gideon, P.; Griffin, M.R. Nonaspirin NSAIDs, cyclooxygenase 2 inhibitors, and the risk for stroke. *Stroke* **2008**, *39*, 2037–2045. [CrossRef]
58. Parkhutik, V.; Lago, A.; Tembl, J.I.; Rubio, C.; Fuset, M.P.; Vallés, J.; Santos, M.T.; Moscardo, A. Influence of COX-inhibiting Analgesics on the Platelet Function of Patients with Subarachnoid Hemorrhage. *J. Stroke Cerebrovasc. Dis.* **2012**, *21*, 755–759. [CrossRef] [PubMed]
59. Park, H.K.; Lee, S.H.; Chu, K.; Roh, J.K. Effects of celecoxib on volumes of hematoma and edema in patients with primary intracerebral hemorrhhage. *J. Neurol. Sci.* **2009**, *279*, 43–46. [CrossRef] [PubMed]
60. Caldwell, B.; Aldington, S.; Weatherall, M.; Shirtcliffe, P.; Beasley, R. Risk of Cardiovascular Events and Celecoxib: A Systematic Review and Meta-Analysis. *J. R. Soc. Med.* **2006**, *99*, 132–140. [CrossRef]
61. Coyle, A.T.; Miggin, S.M.; Kinsella, B.T. Characterization of the 5′ untranslated region of alpha and beta isoforms of the human thromboxane A2 receptor (TP). Differential promoter utilization by the TP isoforms. *Eur. J. Biochem.* **2002**, *269*, 4058–4073. [CrossRef]
62. Davì, G.; Patrono, C. Platelet Activation and Atherothrombosis. *N. Engl. J. Med.* **2007**, *357*, 2482–2494. [CrossRef]
63. Ansar, S.; Larsen, C.; Maddahi, A.; Edvinsson, L. Subarachnoid hemorrhage induces enhanced expression of thromboxane A2 receptors in rat cerebral arteries. *Brain Res.* **2010**, *1316*, 163–172. [CrossRef] [PubMed]
64. Tohgi, H.; Konno, S.; Tamura, K.; Kimura, B.; Kawano, K. Effects of low-to-high doses of aspirin on platelet aggregability and metabolites of thromboxane A2 and prostacyclin. *Stroke* **1992**, *23*, 1400–1403. [CrossRef] [PubMed]
65. Vinge, E.; Brandt, L.; Ljunggren, B.; Andersson, K.E. Thromboxane B2 levels in serum during continous administration of nimodipine to patients with aneurysmal subarachnoid hemorrhage. *Stroke* **1988**, *19*, 644–647. [CrossRef]
66. Collins, T.; Read, M.A.; Neish, A.S.; Whitley, M.Z.; Thanos, D.; Maniatis, T. Transcriptional regulation of endothelial cell adhesion molecules: NF-kappa B and cytokine-inducible enhancers. *FASEB J.* **1995**, *9*, 899–909. [CrossRef] [PubMed]
67. Node, K.; Huo, Y.; Ruan, X.; Yang, B.; Spiecker, M.; Ley, K.; Zeldin, D.C.; Liao, J.K. Anti-inflammatory Properties of Cytochrome P450 Epoxygenase-Derived Eicosanoids. *Science* **1999**, *285*, 1276–1279. [CrossRef]
68. Xiao, L.; Liu, Y.; Wang, N. New paradigms in inflammatory signaling in vascular endothelial cells. *Am. J. Physiol. Circ. Physiol.* **2014**, *306*, H317–H325. [CrossRef]
69. Muldoon, L.L.; Alvarez, J.I.; Begley, D.J.; Boado, R.J.; Del Zoppo, G.J.; Doolittle, N.D.; Engelhardt, B.; Hallenbeck, J.M.; Lonser, R.R.; Ohlfest, J.R.; et al. Immunologic Privilege in the Central Nervous System and the Blood–Brain Barrier. *J. Cereb. Blood Flow Metab.* **2013**, *33*, 13–21. [CrossRef]
70. Siler, D.A.; Berlow, Y.A.; Kukino, A.; Davis, C.M.; Nelson, J.W.; Grafe, M.R.; Ono, H.; Cetas, J.S.; Pike, M.; Alkayed, N.J. Soluble Epoxide Hydrolase in Hydrocephalus, Cerebral Edema, and Vascular Inflammation after Subarachnoid Hemorrhage. *Stroke* **2015**, *46*, 1916–1922. [CrossRef]
71. Greenwood, J.; Etienne-Manneville, S.; Adamson, P.; Couraud, P.-O. Lymphocyte migration into the central nervous system: Implication of ICAM-1 signalling at the blood–brain barrier. *Vasc. Pharmacol.* **2002**, *38*, 315–322. [CrossRef] [PubMed]
72. Laufs, U.; La Fata, V.; Plutzky, J.; Liao, J.K. Upregulation of Endothelial Nitric Oxide Synthase by HMG CoA Reductase Inhibitors. *Circulation* **1998**, *97*, 1129–1135. [CrossRef] [PubMed]
73. McGirt, M.J.; Lynch, J.R.; Parra, A.; Sheng, H.; Pearlstein, R.D.; Laskowitz, D.T.; Pelligrino, D.A.; Warner, D.S. Simvastatin Increases Endothelial Nitric Oxide Synthase and Ameliorates Cerebral Vasospasm Resulting From Subarachnoid Hemorrhage. *Stroke* **2002**, *33*, 2950–2956. [CrossRef]

74. Weitz-Schmidt, G. Statins as anti-inflammatory agents. *Trends Pharmacol. Sci.* **2002**, *23*, 482–487. [CrossRef]
75. McGirt, M.J.; Pradilla, G.; Legnani, F.G.; Thai, Q.-A.; Recinos, P.F.; Tamargo, R.J.; Clatterbuck, R.E. Systemic Administration of Simvastatin after the Onset of Experimental Subarachnoid Hemorrhage Attenuates Cerebral Vasospasm. *Neurosurgery* **2006**, *58*, 945–951. [CrossRef]
76. Vergouwen, M.D.; de Haan, R.J.; Vermeulen, M.; Roos, Y.B. Effect of statin treatment on vasospasm, delayed cerebral ischemia, and functional outcome in patients with aneurysmal subarachnoid hemorrhage: A systematic review and meta-analysis update. *Stroke* **2010**, *41*, e47–e52. [CrossRef]
77. Liu, T.; Zhong, S.; Zhai, Q.; Zhang, X.; Jing, H.; Li, K.; Liu, S.; Han, S.; Li, L.; Shi, X.; et al. Optimal Course of Statins for Patients With Aneurysmal Subarachnoid Hemorrhage: Is Longer Treatment Better? A Meta-Analysis of Randomized Controlled Trials. *Front. Neurosci.* **2021**, *15*, 757505. [CrossRef] [PubMed]
78. Maher, M.; Schweizer, T.A.; Macdonald, R.L. Treatment of Spontaneous Subarachnoid Hemorrhage: Guidelines and Gaps. *Stroke* **2020**, *51*, 1326–1332. [CrossRef] [PubMed]
79. Guan, X.; Wang, Y.; Kai, G.; Zhao, S.; Huang, T.; Li, Y.; Xu, Y.; Zhang, L.; Pang, T. Cerebrolysin Ameliorates Focal Cerebral Ischemia Injury Through Neuroinflammatory Inhibition via CREB/PGC-1α Pathway. *Front. Pharmacol.* **2019**, *10*, 1245. [CrossRef]
80. Muresanu, D.F.; Heiss, W.D.; Hoemberg, V.; Bajenaru, O.; Popescu, C.D.; Vester, J.C.; Rahlfs, V.W.; Doppler, E.; Meier, D.; Moessler, H.; et al. Cerebrolysin and recovery after stroke (CARS): A randomized, placebo-controlled, double-blind, multicenter trial. *Stroke* **2016**, *47*, 151–159. [CrossRef]
81. Xue, L.X.; Zhang, T.; Zhao, Y.W.; Geng, Z.; Chen, J.J.; Chen, H. Efficacy and safety comparison of DL-3-n.butylphtalide and Cerebrolysin: Effects on neurological and behavioral outcomes in acute ischemic stroke. *Exp. Ther. Med.* **2016**, *11*, 2015–2020. [CrossRef]
82. Lang, W.; Stadler, C.H.; Poljakovic, Z.; Fleet, D. The Lyse Study Group. A Prospective, Randomized, Placebo-Controlled, Double-Blind Trial about Safety and Efficacy of Combined Treatment with Alteplase (rt-PA) and Cerebrolysin in Acute Ischaemic Hemispheric Stroke. *Int. J. Stroke* **2012**, *8*, 95–104. [CrossRef]
83. Chang, W.H.; Park, C.H.; Kim, D.Y.; Shin, Y.I.; Ko, M.H.; Lee, A.; Jang, S.Y.; Kim, Y.H. Cerebrolysin combined with rehabilitation promotes motro recovery in patients with severe motor impairment after stroke. *BMC Neurol.* **2016**, *16*, 31. [CrossRef]
84. Gharagozli, K.; Harandi, A.; Houshmand, S.; Akbari, N.; Muresanu, D.; Vester, J.; Winter, S.; Moessler, H. Efficacy and safety of Cerebrolysin treatment in early recovery after acute ischemic stroke: A randomized, placebo-controlled, double-blinded, multicenter clinical trial. *J. Med. Life* **2017**, *10*, 153–160.
85. Rezaei, Y.; Amiri-Nikpour, M.R.; Nazarbaghi, S.; Ahmadi-Salmasi, B.; Mokari, T.; Tahmtan, O. Cerebrolysin effects on neurological outcomes and cerebral blood flow in acute ischemic stroke. *Neuropsychiatr. Dis. Treat.* **2014**, *10*, 2299–2306. [CrossRef]
86. Park, Y.K.; Yi, H.-J.; Choi, K.-S.; Lee, Y.-J.; Kim, D.-W.; Kwon, S.M. Cerebrolysin for the Treatment of Aneurysmal Subarachnoid Hemorrhage in Adults: A Retrospective Chart Review. *Adv. Ther.* **2018**, *35*, 2224–2235. [CrossRef] [PubMed]
87. Rios, C.; Nader-Kawachi, J.; Rodriguez-Payán, A.J.; Nava-Ruiz, C. Neuroprotective effect of dapsone in an occlusive model of focal ischemia in rats. *Brain Res.* **2004**, *999*, 212–215. [CrossRef] [PubMed]
88. Suda, T.; Suzuki, Y.; Matsui, T.; Inoue, T.; Niide, O.; Yoshimaru, T.; Suzuki, H.; Ra, C.; Ochiai, T. Dapsone suppresses human neutrophil superoxide production and elastase release in a calcium-dependent manner. *Br. J. Dermatol.* **2005**, *152*, 887–895. [CrossRef]
89. He, J.; Zhang, X.; He, W.; Xie, Y.; Chen, Y.; Yang, Y.; Chen, R. Neuroprotective effects of zonisamide on cerebral ischemia injury via inhibition of neuronal apoptosis. *Braz. J. Med. Biol. Res.* **2021**, *54*, e10498. [CrossRef] [PubMed]
90. Nader-Kawachi, J.; Góngora-Rivera, F.; Santos-Zambrano, J.; Calzada, P.; Ríos, C. Neuroprotective effect of dapsone in patients with acute ischemic stroke: A pilot study. *Neurol. Res.* **2007**, *29*, 331–334. [CrossRef]
91. Mistry, A.; Mistry, E.A.; Kumar, N.G.; Froehler, M.T.; Fusco, M.R.; Chitale, R.V. Corticosteroids in the Management of Hyponatremia, Hypovolemia, and Vasospasm in Subarachnoid Hemorrhage: A Meta-Analysis. *Cerebrovasc. Dis.* **2016**, *42*, 263–271. [CrossRef]
92. Brown, R.J.; Epling, B.P.; Staff, I.; Fortunato, G.; Grady, J.J.; McCullough, L.D. Polyuria and cerebral vasospasm after aneurysmal subarachnoid hemorrhage. *BMC Neurol.* **2015**, *15*, 201. [CrossRef] [PubMed]
93. Egge, A.; Waterloo, K.; Sjoholm, H.; Solberg, T.; Ingebrigtsen, T.; Romner, B. Prophylactic hyperdynamic postoperative fluid therapy after aneurysmal subarachnoid hemorrhage: A clinical, prospective, randomized, controlled study. *Neurosurgery* **2001**, *49*, 593–605. [PubMed]
94. Lennihan, L.; Mayer, S.A.; Fink, M.E.; Beckford, A.; Paik, M.C.; Zhang, H.; Wu, Y.C.; Klebanoff, L.M.; Raps, E.C.; Solomon, R.A. Effect of hypervolemic therapy on cerebral blood flow after subarachnoid hemorrhage: A randomized controlled trial. *Stroke* **2000**, *31*, 383–391. [CrossRef] [PubMed]
95. Nakagawa, I.; Hironaka, Y.; Nishimura, F.; Takeshima, Y.; Matsuda, R.; Yamada, S.; Motoyama, Y.; Park, Y.-S.; Nakase, H. Early Inhibition of Natriuresis Suppresses Symptomatic Cerebral Vasospasm in Patients with Aneurysmal Subarachnoid Hemorrhage. *Cerebrovasc. Dis.* **2013**, *35*, 131–137. [CrossRef]
96. Miller, B.A.; Turan, N.; Chau, M.; Pradilla, G. Inflammation, vasospasm, and brain injury after subarachnoid hemorrhage. *Biomed. Res. Int.* **2014**, *2014*, 384342. [CrossRef]

97. Chaudhry, S.R.; Stoffel-Wagner, B.; Kinfe, T.M.; Güresir, E.; Vatter, H.; Dietrich, D.; Lamprecht, A.; Muhammad, S. Elevated Systemic IL-6 Levels in Patients with Aneurysmal Subarachnoid Hemorrhage Is an Unspecific Marker for Post-SAH Complications. *Int. J. Mol. Sci.* **2017**, *18*, 2580. [CrossRef]
98. Chyatte, D.; Fode, N.C.R.N.; Nichols, D.A.; Sundt, T.M. Preliminary Report: Effects of High Dose Methylprednisolone on Delayed Cerebral Ischemia in Patients at High Risk for Vasospasm after Aneurysmal Subarachnoid Hemorrhage. *Neurosurgery* **1987**, *21*, 157–160. [CrossRef]
99. McGirt, M.J.; Mavropoulos, J.C.; McGirt, L.Y.; Alexander, M.J.; Friedman, A.H.; Laskowitz, D.T.; Lynch, J.R. Leukcytosis as an independent risk factor for cerebral vasospasm following aneurysmal subarachnoid hemorrhage. *J. Neurosurg.* **2003**, *98*, 1222–1226. [CrossRef]
100. Schürkämper, M.; Medele, R.; Zausinger, S.; Schmid-Elsaesser, R.; Steiger, H.-J. Dexamethasone in the treatment of subarachnoid hemorrhage revisited: A comparative analysis of the effect of the total dose on complications and outcome. *J. Clin. Neurosci.* **2004**, *11*, 20–24. [CrossRef]
101. Güresir, E.; Lampmann, T.; Bele, S.; Czabanka, M.; Czorlich, P.; Gempt, J.; Goldbrunner, R.; Hurth, H.; Hermann, E.; Jabbarli, R.; et al. Fight INflammation to Improve outcome after aneurysmal Subarachnoid HEmorRhage (FINISHER) trial: Study protocol for a randomized controlled trial. *Int. J. Stroke* **2022**, *18*, 242–247. [CrossRef]
102. Brotman, D.J.; Girod, J.P.; Posch, A.; Jani, J.T.; Patel, J.V.; Gupta, M.; Lip, G.Y.; Reddy, S.; Kickler, T.S. Effects of short-term glucocorticoids on hemostatic factors in healthy volunteers. *Thromb. Res.* **2006**, *118*, 247–252. [CrossRef]
103. Isidori, A.M.; Minnetti, M.; Sbardella, E.; Graziadio, C.; Grossman, A.B. Mechanisms in endocrinology: The spectrum of haemostatic abnormalities in glucocorticoid excess and defect. *Eur. J. Endocrinol.* **2015**, *173*, R101–R113. [CrossRef] [PubMed]
104. Ornelas, A.; Zacharias-Millward, N.; Menter, D.G.; Davis, J.S.; Lichtenberger, L.; Hawke, D.; Hawk, E.; Vilar, E.; Bhattacharya, P.; Millward, S. Beyond COX-1: The effects of aspirin on platelet biology and potential mechanisms of chemoprevention. *Cancer Metastasis Rev.* **2017**, *36*, 289–303. [CrossRef] [PubMed]
105. Page, M.J.; McKenzie, J.E.; Bossuyt, P.M.; Boutron, I.; Hoffmann, T.C.; Mulrow, C.D.; Shamseer, L.; Tetzlaff, J.M.; Akl, E.A.; Brennan, S.E.; et al. The PRISMA 2020 statement: An updated guideline for reporting systematic reviews. *BMJ* **2021**, *372*, n71. [CrossRef] [PubMed]

Disclaimer/Publisher's Note: The statements, opinions and data contained in all publications are solely those of the individual author(s) and contributor(s) and not of MDPI and/or the editor(s). MDPI and/or the editor(s) disclaim responsibility for any injury to people or property resulting from any ideas, methods, instructions or products referred to in the content.

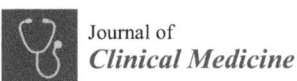

Article

Unruptured Anterior Communicating Artery Aneurysms: Management Strategy and Results of a Single-Center Experience

Katarzyna Wójtowicz [1], Lukasz Przepiorka [1,*], Sławomir Kujawski [2], Andrzej Marchel [1] and Przemysław Kunert [1]

[1] Department of Neurosurgery, Medical University of Warsaw, 02-091 Warsaw, Poland
[2] Department of Exercise Physiology and Functional Anatomy, Ludwik Rydygier Collegium Medicum in Bydgoszcz, Nicolaus Copernicus University in Toruń, 85-077 Bydgoszcz, Poland
* Correspondence: lukaszprzepi@gmail.com; Tel.: +48-22-599-25-75

Abstract: Although anterior communicating artery (AComA) unruptured intracranial aneurysms (UIAs) comprise one of the largest aneurysm subgroups, their complex adjacent neurovasculature and increased risk of rupture impede optimal management. In the present study, we analyzed the results of our diverse strategy in AComA UIAs with the additional goal of assessing the risk of treatment and the incidence of hemorrhage. We analyzed 131 patients, of which each was assessed by a multidisciplinary neurovascular team and assigned to observation (45.8%), endovascular treatment (34.4%) or microsurgery (19.8%). Median aneurysm sizes were 3, 7.2 and 7.75 mm, respectively. In the observation group, four (7.1%) aneurysms (initially <5 mm) grew over a median time of 63.5 months and were treated endovascularly. We found that fewer patients in the observation group were smokers ($p = 0.021$). The aneurysm size ratio was different between the combined treatment versus the observation group ($p < 0.0001$). Noteworthily, there were no hemorrhages in the observational group. Mortality for all patients with available follow-up was 2.4% (3/124) and permanent morbidity was 1.6% (2/124) over a mean follow-up of 64.2 months. These compelling rates refer to a high-risk group with potentially devastating consequences in which we have decreased the annual risk of hemorrhage to 0.14%.

Keywords: unruptured intracranial aneurysms; microsurgery; endovascular; observation; management; anterior communicating artery; morbidity; mortality

1. Introduction

The prevalence of unruptured intracranial aneurysms (UIAs) is estimated at 3.2% [1]. The anterior communicating artery (AComA) region stands out from other anatomical locations due to its congestion of functionally important structures, namely, numerous perforators, and relatively frequent prevalence of AComA UIAs. Additionally, AComA UIAs may exhibit twice the risk of rupture than other UIAs with an annual risk of rupture as high as 2.2% [2,3].

Even though AComA aneurysms comprise the biggest subgroup of all UIAs, their optimal management remains unclear. As with any other UIA, each patient needs to be qualified for observation or treatment. Endovascular techniques and microsurgery are standard methods of treatment, though the choice of which of them for patients qualified for treatment is often subjective.

To overcome this lack of unequivocal management guidelines, numerous scales and algorithms have been designed to facilitate the decision-making process [4–6]. In the present study, we analyze the results of our diverse management strategy in patients with AComA UIAs. We additionally set out to assess the risk of treatment including complications, the immediate and long-term outcomes of the endovascular treatment as well as open surgery.

Moreover, we endeavored to measure the incidence of aneurysmal hemorrhage in each of three management option groups.

2. Materials and Methods

This study was designed as a retrospective, single-center, consecutive case series, undertaken in an academic setting from 2011 to 2021. For each patient, the multidisciplinary team—comprising neurological surgeons and neurointerventional radiologists—qualified patients for observation or treatment. Our management strategy changed over time. At the beginning, it was based on the algorithm published by Chalouhi et al. [7]. Over time, we gradually remodeled the assessment of the risk of hemorrhage according to the PHASES and integrated additional tools as well as the UIATS recommendations [4,5]. When needed, the multidisciplinary team chose the treatment modality. In general, endovascular treatment was the preferred modality for patients qualified for treatment, unless the aneurysm configuration made it particularly hazardous, in which case microsurgery was chosen.

We analyzed our long-term clinical follow-up for all groups. In the observational and endovascular groups, we analyzed radiological outcomes, whereas in the endovascular and microsurgical groups, we analyzed clinical outcomes immediately and at discharge. Clinical outcomes were assessed with the modified Rankin scale (mRS). Good outcomes were defined as an mRS score of 0 to 2, and poor outcomes were defined as an mRS score greater than 2. Neurological deficits were divided into minor (mRS 1 to 2) and major (mRS greater than 2). Deterioration was defined as an increase of at least 1 point in the mRS score. Follow-up information was obtained during routine clinic visits or telephone interviews.

2.1. Follow-Up Algorithm

Patients in the observational group were monitored as follows: outpatient clinic visits with a computed tomography angiography (CTA) or magnetic resonance angiography (MRA) at six months and then once a year thereafter.

In the endovascular group, we routinely perform a posttreatment digital subtraction angiography (DSA) approximately 6 months after the endovascular procedure, and in case of a satisfactory result, this is the last radiological study performed. Subsequent DSAs are performed only when necessary (i.e., incomplete occlusion in the first posttreatment DSA, visible remnant, etc.). We use the Raymond–Roy (RROC) grading scale to assess aneurysm occlusion [8]. As a rule in our institution, we waive routine postoperative vascular imaging (DSA, CTA, and MRA) after microsurgery. From 2018, we started routinely using intraoperative indocyanine green videoangiography to confirm the patency of the arteries and closure of the aneurysm. Prior to that, we performed early postoperative CTA in uncertain cases.

2.2. Statistical Analyses

We performed the Shapiro–Wilk and Levene's tests to examine assumptions of data normality and the equality of variances, respectively. We examined the associations between qualitative variables with the chi-squared or Fisher's exact tests. Differences between two groups were evaluated with the Mann–Whitney U or independent t-tests, depending on the assumptions met. Differences between more than two groups were evaluated with the Kruskal–Wallis H test or one-way ANOVA, depending on the assumptions met. Post hoc comparisons were made using the Dunn test, and values were adjusted for multiple comparisons. All analyses were performed using R [9], and violin graphs were created with the ggstatsplot library [10]. Effect size (ε) and confidence interval [−95%; 95%] from the ggstatsplot library are reported for the Kruskal–Wallis test result. All analyses were performed with a significance level of $\alpha = 0.05$.

3. Results

During the study period 131 patients were diagnosed with 131 UIAs AComA. Initially, 60 cases (45.8%) were classified to the observation group and 71 cases (54.2%) to the treatment group, of which, 45 cases (63.4%) were qualified to endovascular and 26 cases

(36.6%) to microsurgical treatment (Table 1 and Figure 1). After crossovers, we analyzed 64 patients in the observational group, 44 patients in the endovascular treatment group and 25 patients in the microsurgery group. These numbers exceed the total number of patients diagnosed with UIAs AComA. The reason for that is that patients initially observed—until diagnosed with aneurysmal growth—were included in both the observation group (for the whole observation period) and the endovascular group (after qualification for treatment). The demographics and aneurysmal risk factors for each analyzed group are presented in Table 2.

Table 1. Demographics and aneurysmal characteristics of groups of patients as initially assigned. Abbreviations: IA—intracranial aneurysm, SAH—subarachnoid hemorrhage.

Data	Observation Group No. (%)	Endovascular Group No. (%)	Microsurgical Group No. (%)	p
Initial assignment	60 (45.8%)	45 (34.4%)	26 (19.8%)	
Sex				
male	23 (38.3%)	20 (44.44%)	10 (38.46%)	$p = 0.8$
female	37 (61.7%)	25 (55.56%)	16 (61.54%)	
Age, years				$p = 0.1$
median	65	62	57.5	
patients under 40 years old	5 (8.3%)	4 (8.8%)	3 (11.5%)	$p = 0.9$
Family history of SAH or IAs	5 (8.3%)	5 (11.1%)	4 (15.4%)	$p = 0.8$
Previous SAH from another aneurysm	5 (8.3%)	1 (2.2%)	1 (3.8%)	$p = 0.42$
Hypertension	38 (63.3%)	36 (80%)	23 (88.5%)	$p = 0.06$
Smoking	17 (28.3%)	20 (44.4%)	15 (57.7%)	$p = 0.02$
Initial medical condition (mRS)				
0	56 (93.3%)	43 (95.6%)	23 (92%)	
1	2 (3.3%)	1 (2.2%)	1 (4%)	
2	0	0	1 (4%)	
3	1 (1.7%)	1 (2.2%)	0	
4	1 (1.7%)	0	0	
5	0	0	0	
Aneurysm size, mm				
median	3	7.2	7.75	$p < 0.001$
range	1.4–9	2.7–18.9	3.5–25	
Aneurysm size groups				
<5 mm	49 (81.7%)	6 (13.3%)	3 (11.5%)	
5–7 mm	8 (13.3%)	15 (33.3%)	9 (34.6%)	
>7–12 mm	3 (5%)	20 (44.4%)	9 (34.6%)	
>12–25 mm	0	4 (8.9%)	3 (11.5%)	
>25 mm	0	0	2 (7.7%)	
Aspect ratio > 1.6	10 (16.7%)	27 (60%)	11 (42.3%)	$p < 0.0001$
Size ratio > 3	5 (8.3%)	24 (53.3%)	18 (69.2%)	$p < 0.0001$
Multilobulated	5 (8.3%)	17 (37.8%)	1 (3.8%)	$p < 0.001$
Multiple	22 (36.7%)	19 (42.2%)	10 (38.5%)	$p < 0.9$
Symptomatic aneurysms	0	0	2 (8%): 1 (4%) visual symptom and 1 (4%) seizure	$p < 0.04$

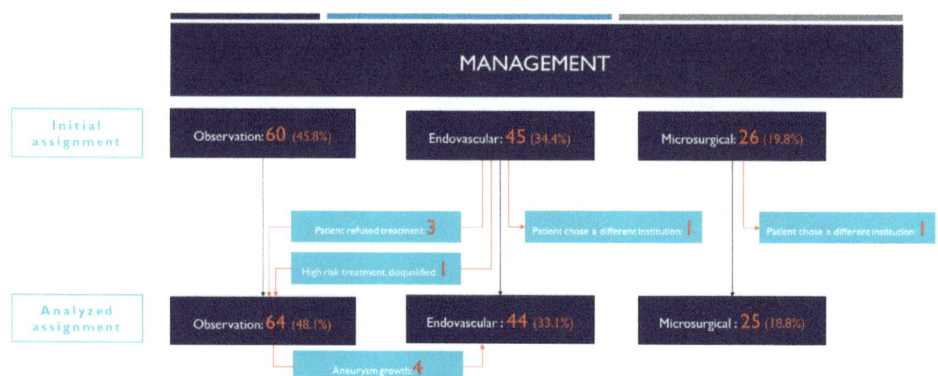

Figure 1. Management of patients with unruptured anterior communicating artery aneurysms as they were initially assigned and then analyzed in our study.

Table 2. Demographics and aneurysmal characteristics of analyzed groups of patients.

Data	Observation Group No. (%)	Endovascular Group No. (%)	Microsurgical Group No. (%)	p
Analyzed assignment *	64 (48.1%)	44 (33.1%)	25 (18.8%)	
Sex				
male	24 (37.5%)	19 (43.2%)	10 (40%)	p = 0.839
female	40 (62.5%)	25 (56.8%)	15 (60%)	
Age, years				
median	65.5	62	56	p = 0.072
patients under 40 years old	5 (7.8%)	4 (9%)	3 (12%)	
Family history of SAH or IAs	5 (7.8%)	5 (11.4%)	4 (16%)	p = 0.675
Previous SAH from another aneurysm	0	0	1 (4%)	p = 0.606
Hypertension	42 (65.6%)	34 (77.3%)	23 (92%)	p = 0.062
Smoking	17 (26.6%)	19 (43.2%)	14 (56%)	p = 0.024
Initial medical condition (mRS)				
0	59 (92.2%)	42 (95.5%)	23 (92%)	
1	2 (3.1%)	2 (4.5%)	1 (4%)	
2	0	0	1 (4%)	
3	2 (3.1%)	0	0	
4	1 (1.6%)	0	0	
5	0	0	0	
Aneurysm size, mm				
median	3	7	8	p < 0.001
range	1.4–9	2.7–18.9	3.5–25	
Aneurysm size groups				
<5 mm	49 (76.6%)	6 (13.6%)	2 (8%)	
5–7 mm	10 (15.6%)	16 (36.4%)	6 (36%)	
>7–12 mm	5 (7.8%)	19 (43.2%)	12 (48%)	
>12–25 mm	0	3 (6.8%)	3 (12%)	
>25 mm	0	0	2 (8%)	
Aspect ratio > 1.6	12 (18.75%)	27 (61.4%)	11 (44%)	p < 0.0001
Size ratio > 3	8 (12.5%)	22 (50%)	19 (76%)	p < 0.0001
Multilobulated	6 (9.4%)	18 (40.9%)	1 (4%)	p < 0.001
Multiple aneurysms	23 (35.9%)	20 (45.5%)	9 (36%)	p = 0.572
Symptomatic aneurysms	0	0	2 (8%): 1 (4%) visual symptom and 1 (4%) seizure	p = 0.034

* Sum of analyzed patients exceeds total number of patients—an explanation is provided in the text. Abbreviations: IA—intracranial aneurysm, SAH—subarachnoid hemorrhage.

3.1. Observation Group

3.1.1. Assignment

Sixty patients were initially qualified for the conservative management specified earlier. Additionally, four patients initially assigned to the endovascular treatment group were moved to the observational group. Three patients refused endovascular treatment. In one case during diagnostic DSA, the risk of an endovascular treatment had been assessed as high, and treatment was not undertaken. For that reason, the analyzed observational group comprised 64 subjects. Significantly fewer patients in the observation group were smokers (chi-square test, $p = 0.021$). The aneurysm size ratio was significantly different between the combined treatment groups versus the observation group (Kruskal–Wallis $p < 0.0001$, $\varepsilon = 0.45$ [0.33; 1]). Post hoc tests showed that the size ratio was significantly smaller in the observational group in comparison to the endovascular and microsurgery groups (both $p < 0.0001$) (Figure 2A).

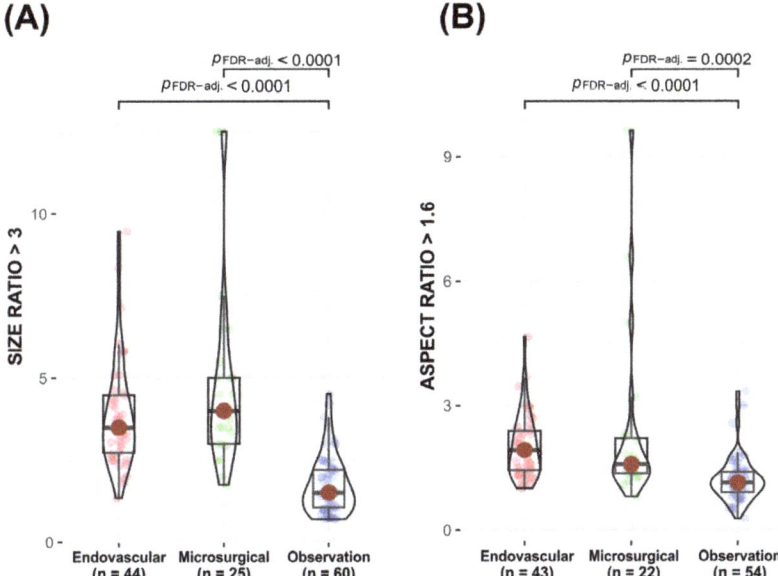

Figure 2. Comparison of size ratio (**A**) and aspect ratio (**B**) between endovascular, microsurgical and observation groups. Red dots and horizontal black lines inside the box indicate median value. Magenta dots in endovascular, green dots in microsurgical and blue in observation groups denote the results of individual patients. The shape of the violin graph indicates the distribution of results.

In addition, the aneurysm aspect ratio was significantly different between examined groups (Kruskal–Wallis $p < 0.0001$, $\varepsilon = 0,31$ [0.19; 1]). Post hoc tests showed that the aspect ratio was significantly higher in the endovascular and microsurgery groups than in the observational group ($p < 0.0001$ and $p = 0.0002$, respectively) (Figure 2B).

Subsequently, during the observation period, in four cases (6.25%), we observed aneurysmal growth, and these patients were qualified for endovascular treatment. These aneurysms were not significantly different from the remaining aneurysms in statistical analysis. Of note is that these aneurysms—up till their growth—were included in the observation group analysis. In the observation group, three patients (4.67%) had poor initial neurological condition (mRS 3 or more). These were caused by unrelated conditions such as ischemic stroke (n = 2) and lower extremity peripheral artery disease (n = 1).

3.1.2. Radiological Outcomes

Radiological follow-up data were available for 56 patients (87.5%). During the observation period, four (7.1%) aneurysms grew and were treated endovascularly. The median time to the aneurysm growth was 63.5 months (range: 54–73 months); in each case, the initial aneurysm size was under 5 mm. For the remaining (in other words, stable) 52 (92.9%) aneurysms, the mean radiological follow-up was 60.7 months (range: 5–184). The median follow-up for aneurysms under observation, including aneurysms that eventually grew, was 60.9 (range: 5–184).

3.1.3. Clinical Outcomes

Clinical outcomes were available for 63 patients (98.4%); however, 1 patient was lost to the long-term follow-up. Mean clinical follow-up was 71.5 months (range: 7–187). There were no subarachnoid hemorrhages (SAH) or other symptoms of UIA during this period. Five patients (7.9%) died because of unrelated reasons.

3.2. Endovascular Treatment

3.2.1. Assignment

The endovascular group primarily included 45 patients. Of these, one patient (2.2%) chose treatment in another institution, and three patients (6.67%) refused endovascular treatment. In the remaining case (2.2%), after a diagnostic DSA, due to the expected high risk of treatment, an endovascular procedure was not initiated. Moreover, four patients (6.7%) from the observational group were diagnosed with aneurysmal growth and qualified for treatment. No significant differences were found in the size, aspect ratio and size ratio between those four patients and the rest of the endovascular group (all $p > 0.05$). Finally, after relocations, 44 patients were treated endovascularly.

The following techniques were used: coiling alone in 59.1% of cases, coiling with stent in 20.5%, coiling with flow-diverting devices in 11.4% and flow-diverting alone in 9.1% of cases. One case (2.3%) required two-staged treatment.

In total, 45 endovascular procedures were performed to treat 44 aneurysms. The intraprocedural complication rate was 17.8% (eight cases), of which 75% (six cases) were asymptomatic. Coil protrusion to the artery occurred in 8.9% of cases (n = 4), after which stent deployment was required. The rate of vasospasm was 2.2%. The intraprocedural rupture rate for all endovascular procedures was 6.7% (three cases).

3.2.2. Clinical Outcomes

On the first postprocedural day, we observed deterioration in five cases (11.1%). In three of these cases, these were minor; in the other two cases, there were major deficits. Deteriorations were caused by ischemic stroke in two cases, which was confirmed by diffusion-weighted imaging (DWI) magnetic resonance (MR). In two other cases, worsening was caused by an intraprocedural hemorrhage (one was an aneurysmal intraoperative rupture, and the second, more serious, was due to an injury of the A2 segment of anterior cerebral artery). A patient with a major deficit due to an intraprocedural hemorrhage and anterior cerebral artery injury died during hospitalization. There were no intraprocedural complications or ischemia in the postoperative MR in the remaining one patient.

At their discharge from hospital, the neurological status of 41 patients (93.2%) was stable, with their mRS scores as before the treatment; 2 patients (4.5%) were discharged in a worse neurological status due to a new, minor deficit in each case. At discharge from hospital, procedure-related permanent morbidity and mortality rates were 4.5% and 2.3%, respectively. Clinical follow-up data were lost for one patient. Four patients died: one during hospitalization, one due to hemorrhage from the treated aneurysm 57 months after treatment and two due to unrelated reasons. There was one hemorrhage for 186.3 patient years.

3.2.3. Radiological Outcomes

Complete obliteration at the time of treatment was achieved for 38 (86.4%) aneurysms. One patient died shortly after the treatment (see above) and three patients were lost to follow-up. For the remaining 40 patients, the median radiological follow-up was 7.25 months (range: 3–14). The complete occlusion rate was 90%, and the near-complete occlusion (visible neck remnant) rate was 5%, while the dome remnant rate was 5%. Of the two aneurysms with dome remnants, one required retreatment, and the other was left untreated and remained under observation due to a high risk of retreatment. Aneurysms with neck remnants (5%) remained under further observation.

In the statistical analysis, aneurysms with near-complete occlusion and aneurysms with dome remnants were significantly bigger (aneurysm size, mm (median (interquartile range)): 10.9 (2.97) vs. 6.72 (3.09), $p = 0.009$; size ratio > 3:4.66 (1.72) vs. 2.83 (1.33), $p = 0.01$; no significant differences in aspect ratio > 1.6) as compared to the completely occluded aneurysms.

Ultimately, 23 patients (52%) patients had a repeated long-term DSA in a mean follow-up of 37.6 months. Recanalization of four previously occluded aneurysms (17.4%) was demonstrated. These patients exhibited more frequent hypertension (Fisher's exact test $p = 0.03$) and multiple aneurysms (Fisher's exact test $p = 0.04$). In long-term follow-up, two aneurysms with neck remnants had complete occlusion without additional treatment. Additionally, complete occlusion was achieved in the retreatment case.

3.3. Microsurgical Group

3.3.1. Assignment

Initially, 26 patients (19.8%) were qualified for elective microsurgery. Of these, 1 patient chose a different institution for treatment, hence, in the final assignment of microsurgery, there were 25 patients. When compared with other groups in our study, these aneurysms caused the mass effect significantly more often (Fisher's exact test $p = 0.04$).

3.3.2. Postoperative Complications

On the postoperative day one, deterioration was noted in seven patients (28%). In one case, the postoperative deficit was temporary. Deteriorations were caused by an ischemic stroke recognizable in CT in six cases (24%). Additionally, one of these patients (4%) had a postoperative epidural hematoma. In the remaining one case (4%), the cause of neurological deterioration was not found. Median aneurysmal size in patients who deteriorated was 7 mm (range: 5–13 mm).

3.3.3. Clinical Outcomes

At discharge from hospital, 19 patients (76%) were stable with their mRS scores as before the treatment. Almost a quarter of patients deteriorated, including five minor deficits (20%) and one major deficit (4%). The patient with a major deficit died one month after the surgery due to medical complications that were a consequence of a neurosurgical treatment.

Long-term clinical follow-up was available for 21 patients (84%), while 4 patients (16%) were lost to long-term follow-up. Mean follow-up was 63 months (range 1–123). Out of six patients (24%) with postoperative deterioration, three patients improved, one patient died (see above), one patient was lost to the follow-up and one patient exhibited permanent deterioration. There was no hemorrhage from the treated aneurysms. Overall mortality for this group was 4.8%, and permanent morbidity (mRS 1) was 4.8%.

3.4. Overall Results

Mortality for all patients (observed, treated endovascularly and treated microsurgically) with available follow-up was 2.4% (3/124), and permanent morbidity was 1.6% (2/124) over a mean follow-up of 64.2 months.

4. Discussion

In this study we presented our management strategy with AComA UIAs and analyzed their treatment results. We focused exclusively on AComA aneurysms because their increased risk of rupture makes them distinct from other UIAs [11]. Management of patients with AComA UIAs still poses a considerable challenge. Treatment of UIAs is intended to prevent SAH, but it involves a substantial risk of morbidity and mortality. At the beginning, in our decision-making process, we followed the algorithm published by Chalouhi et al. [7]. Subsequently, we introduced additional tools: PHASES and the UIATS system score. Applying these scales did not simplify the decision-making process; their recommendations often differed. Additionally, in 43.5% of cases, UIATS suggestions were not definitive. According to the most recent European recommendations, the indications for treatment are even more limited [12]. Even though our management was tailored for each individual case, some general trends emerged and will be discussed below.

4.1. Observational Group

Morphological features of aneurysms, such as their size, size ratio and aspect ratio, were significantly smaller in the observational group. Conversely, patients in the treatment group were significantly more often smokers. As a result of our strategy, there were no intracranial hemorrhages or neurological deteriorations caused by aneurysm in the observational group.

4.2. Endovascular Group

In the endovascular group, procedure-related mortality (that was a consequence of the provided treatment) and permanent morbidity were 2.3%. Morbidity in our series is lower, while the mortality is comparable to that from the meta-analysis of the endovascular treatment of AComA aneurysms by Fang et al. in 2014 [13]. In that study, permanent morbidity was 8% (95% CI 3–20%) for AComA UIAs, and the procedure-related mortality was 2% (95% CI 1–9%) for AComA UIAs. The rate of hemorrhage was 2.3% in our series and is comparable to the meta-analysis results by Fang et al. (2%, 95% CI 0–6%) [13]. In that study, the retreatment rate was 3%, compared to 5% in our series.

In our study, the long-term complete and near-complete occlusion rates were 90% and 95%, respectively, which is similar to what Fang et al. found in their meta-analysis, i.e., 90% for both complete and near-complete occlusions.

A systematic analysis by O'Neill et al. presents data separately for coiling and stent-assisted coiling. Good clinical outcomes were achieved in 99.2% and 92.1% for these two treatment modalities, while treatment-related mortality was 0 and 1.1%, respectively [14]. There were no SAHs from the treated aneurysms in either endovascular treatment technique. Retreatment rates were 4.9% and 6.8%, for coiling and stent-assisted coiling, respectively. All these results are similar to those obtained in our series.

4.3. Microsurgical Group

Morbidity and mortality in our microsurgical group were 4.7% and 4.7% respectively. In the review of the literature by Nussbaum, 3.3% of microsurgically treated patients did not achieve a good clinical outcome, while the mortality rate was 0.3% [15]. The mortality rate in our study is higher (4.7%), but it refers to a single patient in a comparatively small group (n = 25). This patient had an aneurysm that was not amenable to endovascular techniques and had a high risk of rupture. Similarly, the majority of microsurgically treated aneurysms had complex anatomy, and endovascular treatment of these aneurysms was evaluated as too risky.

The higher risk of clipping may be related to a decreasing volume of patients treated microsurgically, which imperils the opportunity to develop, improve and sustain high operative abilities.

4.4. Final Comments

The observation of aneurysms did not expose patients to hemorrhage and at the same time avoided the risk of treatment, possibly reducing the mortality and morbidity in the whole group. On the other hand, despite the risk of morbidity of endovascular and microsurgical treatment in our material being 2.3% and 4.7%, respectively, the cumulative morbidity risk for the whole study population was lower, at 1.6%. Ultimately, it appears beneficial to observe AComA UIAs whenever reasonable and—when treatment is warranted—diversify preventive aneurysm repair modalities.

In a meta-analysis of the natural history of AComA UIAs, Mira et al. estimated the annual risk of rupture at 2.2% [2]. Yet, in our study, with 690.15 patient years of follow-up (129 patients and 5.35 years) and one case of SAH, we managed to decrease this number to the 0.14% annual risk of rupture.

Based on our experience, we conjecture that evaluating each AComA UIA in a multidisciplinary team, with a preference to observe whenever possible and reasonable, may be of benefit. Prior to such evaluation a patient should be carefully evaluated using all available UIA scales (PHASES, UIATS, and ISUIA).

4.5. Limitations

Our study is limited by its retrospective nature and small sample size. Additionally, our multidisciplinary team evaluates many patients from outside hospitals. Most of these patients, when qualified for observation, are not followed in our institution, and thus, such patients were not included in our database. As a result, there is an inflated portion of treated patients, relative to the whole study group, whereas the patients in the observational group constitute only a fraction of patients actually surveilled in our outpatient clinics.

Finally, our management strategy changed over time according to updated guidelines and risk calculators and is not homogenous for the evaluated patients.

5. Conclusions

Using diversified management of AComA UIAs, we have decreased the annual risk of SAH to 0.14% at the expense of 2.4% mortality and 1.6% permanent minor deficit rates. Noteworthily, there were no hemorrhages in the observational group. The morbidity and mortality in AComA UIAs are compelling, but these refer to a high-risk group with potentially devastating consequences.

Author Contributions: Conceptualization, P.K., A.M. and K.W.; methodology, P.K., L.P., S.K., K.W. and A.M.; software, S.K.; validation, P.K., L.P. and K.W.; formal analysis, P.K., L.P., K.W. and S.K.; investigation, K.W., S.K. and A.M.; resources, K.W., L.P. and A.M.; data curation, K.W. and L.P.; writing—original draft preparation, K.W.; writing—review and editing, L.P. and P.K.; visualization, K.W.; supervision, P.K.; project administration, L.P. All authors have read and agreed to the published version of the manuscript.

Funding: This research received no external funding.

Institutional Review Board Statement: This study was conducted in accordance with the Declaration of Helsinki and approved by the Bioethics Committee of the Medical University of Warsaw.

Informed Consent Statement: Patient consent was waived by the Bioethics Committee of the Medical University of Warsaw due to the retrospective character of the study and participants' anonymity.

Data Availability Statement: The data presented in this study are available on request from the corresponding author after acceptance of all the co-authors.

Acknowledgments: The authors would like to thank Andrew Tuson for his language editing help in preparing the manuscript.

Conflicts of Interest: The authors declare no conflict of interest.

References

1. Vlak, M.H.; Algra, A.; Brandenburg, R.; Rinkel, G.J. Prevalence of unruptured intracranial aneurysms, with emphasis on sex, age, comorbidity, country, and time period: A systematic review and meta-analysis. *Lancet Neurol.* **2011**, *10*, 626–636. [CrossRef] [PubMed]
2. Mira, J.M.S.; Costa, F.A.D.O.; Horta, B.L.; Fabião, O.M. Risk of rupture in unruptured anterior communicating artery aneurysms: Meta-analysis of natural history studies. *Surg. Neurol.* **2006**, *66* (Suppl. S3), S12–S19, discussion S19. [CrossRef] [PubMed]
3. Juvela, S. Outcome of Patients with Multiple Intracranial Aneurysms after Subarachnoid Hemorrhage and Future Risk of Rupture of Unruptured Aneurysm. *J. Clin. Med.* **2021**, *10*, 1712. [CrossRef] [PubMed]
4. Etminan, N.; Brown, R.D.; Beseoglu, K.; Juvela, S.; Raymond, J.; Morita, A.; Torner, J.C.; Derdeyn, C.P.; Raabe, A.; Mocco, J.; et al. The unruptured intracranial aneurysm treatment score. *Neurology* **2015**, *85*, 881–889. [CrossRef] [PubMed]
5. Greving, J.P.; Wermer, M.J.; Brown, R.D.; Morita, A.; Juvela, S.; Yonekura, M.; Ishibashi, T.; Torner, J.C.; Nakayama, T.; Rinkel, G.J.; et al. Development of the PHASES score for prediction of risk of rupture of intracranial aneurysms: A pooled analysis of six prospective cohort studies. *Lancet Neurol.* **2014**, *13*, 59–66. [CrossRef] [PubMed]
6. Thompson, B.G.; Brown, R.D., Jr.; Amin-Hanjani, S.; Broderick, J.P.; Cockroft, K.M.; Connolly, E.S., Jr.; Duckwiler, G.R.; Harris, C.C.; Howard, V.J.; Johnston, S.C.; et al. Guidelines for the Management of Patients with Unruptured Intracranial Aneurysms: A Guideline for Healthcare Professionals from the American Heart Association/American Stroke Association. *Stroke* **2015**, *46*, 2368–2400. [CrossRef] [PubMed]
7. Chalouhi, N.; Dumont, A.S.; Randazzo, C.; Tjoumakaris, S.; Gonzalez, L.F.; Rosenwasser, R.; Jabbour, P. Management of incidentally discovered intracranial vascular abnormalities. *Neurosurg. Focus* **2011**, *31*, E1. [CrossRef] [PubMed]
8. Roy, D.; Milot, G.; Raymond, J. Endovascular Treatment of Unruptured Aneurysms. *Stroke* **2001**, *32*, 1998–2004. [CrossRef] [PubMed]
9. R Core Team. *R: A Language and Environment for Statistical Computing*; R Foundation for Statistical Computing: Vienna, Austria, 2021. Available online: https://www.R-project.org/ (accessed on 5 October 2022).
10. Patil, I. Visualizations with statistical details: The 'ggstatsplot' approach. *J. Open Source Softw.* **2021**, *6*, 3167. [CrossRef]
11. Lu, H.T.; Tan, H.Q.; Gu, B.X.; Li, M.H. Risk factors for multiple intracranial aneurysms rupture: A retrospective study. *Clin. Neurol. Neurosurg.* **2013**, *115*, 690–694. [CrossRef] [PubMed]
12. Etminan, N.; de Sousa, D.A.; Tiseo, C.; Bourcier, R.; Desal, H.; Lindgren, A.; Koivisto, T.; Netuka, D.; Peschillo, S.; Lémeret, S.; et al. European Stroke Organisation (ESO) guidelines on management of unruptured intracranial aneurysms. *Eur. Stroke J.* **2022**, *7*, LXXXI-CVI. [CrossRef] [PubMed]
13. Fang, S.; Brinjikji, W.; Murad, M.H.; Kallmes, D.F.; Cloft, H.J.; Lanzino, G. Endovascular treatment of anterior communicating artery aneurysms: A systematic review and meta-analysis. *AJNR Am. J. Neuroradiol.* **2014**, *35*, 943–947. [CrossRef] [PubMed]
14. O'Neill, A.H.; Chandra, R.V.; Lai, L.T. Safety and effectiveness of microsurgical clipping, endovascular coiling, and stent assisted coiling for unruptured anterior communicating artery aneurysms: A systematic analysis of observational studies. *J. Neurointerv. Surg.* **2017**, *9*, 761–765. [CrossRef] [PubMed]
15. Nussbaum, E.S.; Touchette, J.C.; Madison, M.T.; Goddard, J.K.; Lassig, J.P.; Nussbaum, L.A. Microsurgical Treatment of Unruptured Anterior Communicating Artery Aneurysms: Approaches and Outcomes in a Large Contemporary Series and Review of the Literature. *Oper. Neurosurg.* **2020**, *19*, 678–690. [CrossRef] [PubMed]

Disclaimer/Publisher's Note: The statements, opinions and data contained in all publications are solely those of the individual author(s) and contributor(s) and not of MDPI and/or the editor(s). MDPI and/or the editor(s) disclaim responsibility for any injury to people or property resulting from any ideas, methods, instructions or products referred to in the content.

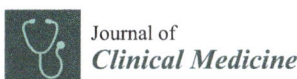 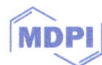

Article

Retrospective Application of Risk Scores to Unruptured Anterior Communicating Artery Aneurysms

Katarzyna Wójtowicz [1,*], Lukasz Przepiorka [1], Sławomir Kujawski [2], Edyta Maj [3], Andrzej Marchel [1] and Przemysław Kunert [1]

1. Department of Neurosurgery, Medical University of Warsaw, 02-097 Warsaw, Poland; amarchel@wum.edu.pl (A.M.); pkunert@wp.pl (P.K.)
2. Department of Exercise Physiology and Functional Anatomy, Ludwik Rydygier Collegium Medicum in Bydgoszcz, Nicolaus Copernicus University in Toruń, 85-077 Bydgoszcz, Poland
3. Second Department of Clinical Radiology, Medical University of Warsaw, 02-097 Warsaw, Poland; em26@wp.pl
* Correspondence: kasia-wojtowicz@wp.pl; Tel.: +48-(51)-7266393

Abstract: Background: Treatment decisions for unruptured intracranial aneurysms (UIAs) pose a challenge for neurosurgeons, prompting the development of clinical scales assessing hemorrhage risk to provide management guidance. This study compares recommendations from the PHASES and UIA treatment scores (UIATS) applied to anterior communicating artery (AComA) UIAs against real-world management. Methods: While UIATS recommends management, for PHASES, an aneurysm with score of 10 or more was considered "high-risk". Analysis involved assessing the concordance in each group alongside comparison to real-word management. Results: Among 129 patients, 46.5% were observed and 53.5% were treated. PHASES scores were significantly higher in the treatment group ($p = 0.00002$), and UIATS recommendations correlated with real-world decisions ($p < 0.001$). We observed no difference in the frequencies of UIATS recommendations between high- and low-risk groups. When comparing the UIATS and PHASES, 33% of high-risk aneurysms received a UIATS conservative management recommendation. In 39% of high-risk aneurysms, the UIATS recommendation was not definitive. Conversely, 27% of low-risk aneurysms obtained a UIATS UIA repair recommendation. Overall, concordance between PHASES and UIATS was 32%. Conclusions: Significant discordance in therapeutic suggestions underscores the predominant influence of center experience and individual assessments. Future studies should refine and validate decision-making strategies, potentially exploring alternative applications or developing tailored scales.

Keywords: unruptured intracranial aneurysm; anterior communicating artery; UIATS; PHASES; concordance

1. Introduction

With the heightened availability and improved precision of diagnostic imaging, in recent years there has been a notable surge in the detection rate of asymptomatic unruptured intracranial aneurysms (UIAs), particularly among elderly patients [1]. This trend is accompanied by a noteworthy inclination to qualify smaller aneurysms for treatment in older patient cohorts. Presumably, this shift in clinical practice is influenced by the advancing safety profile of aneurysm treatment modalities [2,3].

Nevertheless, navigating the decision of whether to treat a UIA presents a challenging dilemma for neurosurgeons worldwide, as well as remaining an ever-present concern in their daily practice. Consequently, several scales have been developed to assess the risk of hemorrhage and offer treatment recommendations. A number of studies have analyzed the usefulness of these scales in predicting the risk of hemorrhage in populations with ruptured intracranial aneurysms, and they show that a large percentage of ruptured aneurysms would have been assigned as low risk aneurysms pre-rupture [4–7].

In this evolving landscape of UIA management, anterior communicating artery (AComA) UIAs stand out. Their distinctive features include high prevalence, proximity to functionally vital structures, and a speculated increased risk of rupture. The aim of this study is to compare management recommendations for AComA UIAs specifically, evaluate different protocols, and compare them with each other and to real-life management of AComA UIAs in a single institution.

2. Materials and Methods

This study is a retrospective evaluation of patients with AComA UIAs who were observed or treated. These patients, including their follow-ups and complications, have already been extensively described in our previous study [8]. In this paper, we applied PHASES and UIATS in comparison to real-life management at a single institution [9,10].

We analyzed the concordance of these scales in each group and compared them to our management. We analyzed a variety of demographics and aneurysm factors to find the differences between the subgroups of different recommendations. The recommendations from UIATS are categorized as either definitive ('UIA repair', i.e., treatment or 'conservative management', i.e., observation) or non-definitive ('the recommendation is not definitive').

This paper will interchangeably refer to recommendations derived from UIA clinical scales and real-world management. To ensure clarity throughout the text, specific terms will be introduced and utilized consistently. We will refer to the real-world aneurysm cohorts as belonging to either the 'treatment' or 'observation' group. Regarding UIATS recommendations, the terms 'UIA repair' or 'conservative management' will be used, as described in the original paper. For the PHASES scale, which assesses the 5-year hemorrhage risk, a score of 10 or more assigned to the aneurysm was considered high-risk, as proposed by Stumpo et al. [11]. Accordingly, whenever the terms 'high-risk' or 'low-risk' aneurysm are utilized in this paper, they will correspond to the PHASES score interpretation.

Statistical Analysis

We performed the Shapiro-Wilk and Levene's tests to examine the assumptions of data normality and the equality of variances, respectively. We examined the associations between qualitative variables with the Chi-squared and Fisher's exact tests. The Chi-square Goodness of Fit test was used to summarize the discrepancy between observed values and expected values. Differences between the two groups were assessed using either the Mann-Whitney U test or independent t-tests, depending on whether assumptions were met. We reported p-values both before and after false discovery rate (FDR) correction. Differences between more than two groups were evaluated with the Kruskal-Wallis H test or one-way ANOVA, depending on whether assumptions were met. Post-hoc comparisons were made using the Dunn test, and p-values were adjusted for multiple comparisons. All analyses were performed using jamovi, which is a graphical user interface for R and violin graphs, which were created using the ggstatsplot library [12–14]. Effect size (ε) and confidence interval [−95%; 95%] from the ggstatsplot library are reported for Kruskal-Wallis test results. All analyses were performed with a significance level of $\alpha = 0.05$.

To mitigate potential high correlation between PHASES and age, as well as UIATS and age, we avoided including these variables as predictors in the same model. Instead, we independently considered age, PHASES, and UIATS in separate models, allowing a distinct assessment of their contributions to our analyses.

3. Results

In our series of 129 patients with AComA UIAs, 46.5% (60) of patients remained under observation and 53.5% (69) were qualified for treatment.

3.1. PHASES Scores and Real-World Management Decisions

There were 111 (86%) AComA aneurysms classified as low-risk (score < 10) and 18 (14%) classified as high-risk (score ≥ 10), according to the PHASES scores.

The PHASES scores were significantly higher in the group qualified for treatment [median ± interquartile range (IQR) was 8 ± 5 in the treatment group vs. 5 ± 1 in the observation group, $p = 0.00002$, Table 1]. Figure 1 presents the distribution of treated and observed AComA aneurysms according to their PHASES scores.

Table 1. PHASES scores in patients with unruptured anterior communicating artery aneurysms who were under observation or were qualified for treatment.

Group	n	PHASES Scores	
		Median	Range
Treatment	69	8	4–15
Observation	60	5	4–9

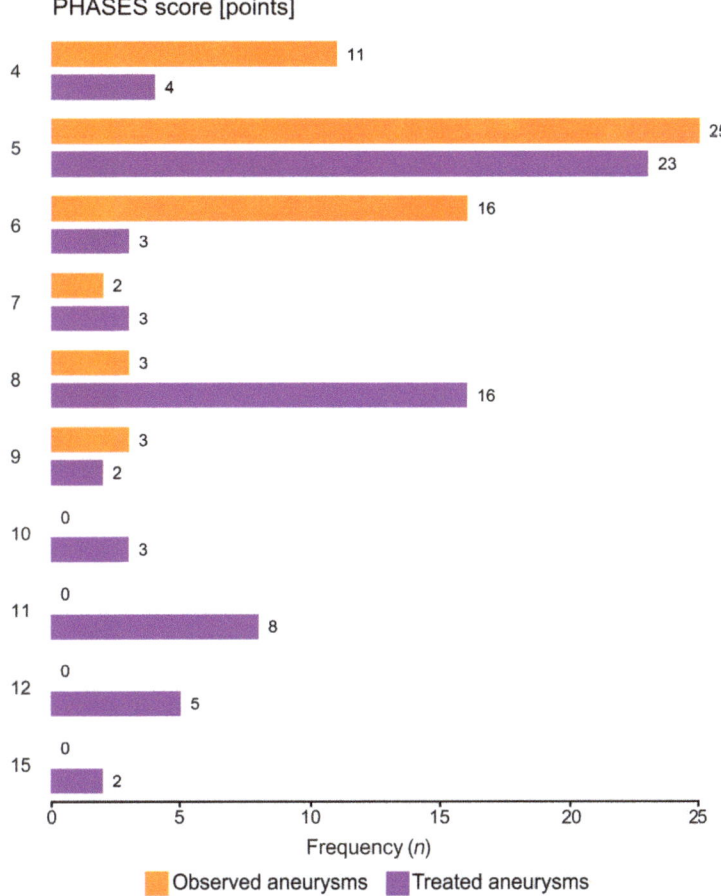

Figure 1. Distribution of PHASES scores across treated and observed unruptured anterior communicating artery aneurysms. Orange—observed aneurysms, violet—treated aneurysms.

3.2. UIATS and Real-World Management Decisions

In accordance with UIATS, UIA repair was recommended for 27% (35) of patients and conservative management for 32% (41) of patients, while the recommendation remained not definitive for 37% (48) of individuals. In five cases, our data was insufficient to calculate UIATS. Patients under observation more frequently received an UIATS conservative management recommendation and, correspondingly, patients who qualified for treatment more frequently received a UIATS UIA repair recommendation (Chi-square test, $p < 0.001$, Table 2). A significant association was identified between UIATS recommendations for UIA repair or conservative management and real-world decisions (Fisher's exact test, $p < 0.001$).

Table 2. UIATS recommendations for patients with unruptured anterior communicating artery aneurysms who were under observation or qualified for treatment. UIA—unruptured intracranial aneurysm.

Group	Recommendation According to UIATS			No Data
	UIA Repair	Conservative Management	Not Definitive	
Observation, $n = 60$	6 (10%)	28 (47%)	21 (35%)	5 (8%)
Treatment, $n = 69$	29 (42%)	13 (19%)	27 (39%)	0

3.3. UIATS Recommendations against PHASES Scores

We observed no difference in the frequencies of UIATS recommendations between high and low-risk groups, as interpreted by PHASES (Table 3, for details please refer to Supplementary Table S1).

Table 3. A comparative analysis of aneurysm evaluations according to PHASES and UIATS recommendations. Aneurysms with PHASES score of 10 and more were classified as high-risk. UIA—unruptured intracranial aneurysm.

PHASES Interpretation of an Aneurysm	Recommendation According to UIATS			Chi-Square Goodness of Fit p-Value
	UIA Repair	Conservative Management	Not Definitive	
Low-risk	30 (28%)	35 (33%)	41 (39%)	0.424
High-risk	5 (28%)	6 (33%)	7 (39%)	0.846

In the entire cohort, PHASES scores were not significantly different in relation to any UIATS recommendation (Chi-squared Kruskal-Wallis = 4.91, $p = 0.086$, Figure 2).

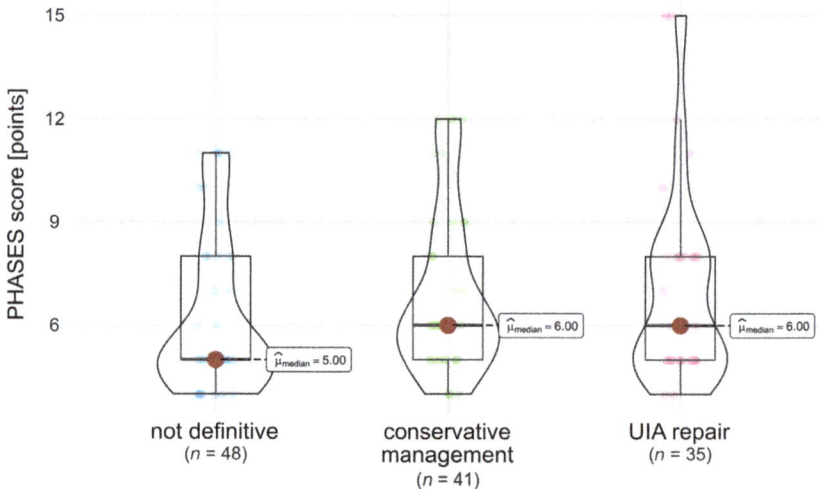

Figure 2. Comparison of PHASES scores in relation to the UIATS recommendation across the whole cohort. A dark red dot denotes the median value, while smaller dots indicate values of individual patients.

In the subgroup of aneurysms with a definitive recommendation, UIATS recommended conservative management for 55% (6) of high-risk and for 54% (35) of low-risk aneurysms, according to PHASES score interpretation. Likewise, in the subgroup with a UIATS definitive recommendation, UIA repair was recommended for 46% (30) of low-risk and for 45% (5) of high-risk aneurysms, as per PHASES score interpretation (chi-squared p-value 0.97).

3.4. Observation Group

PHASES scores in the group of 60 patients under observation ranged from 4 to 9, and no high-risk aneurysms (according to PHASES interpretation) were identified. In this group, UIATS recommended UIA repair for 11% (6) of patients and conservative management for 51% (28) of patients, while 38% (21) of patients lacked a specific recommendation (i.e., the UIATS recommendation was not definitive).

Among patients under observation, PHASES scores were significantly different between subgroups based on UIATS recommendation [Chi-squared Kruskal-Wallis = 6.35, p = 0.042, $\varepsilon 2$ = 0.12 (0.02; 1)]. The subgroup with a UIATS conservative management recommendation had significantly higher PHASES scores when compared against patients with 'not definitive' recommendations (p = 0.035, Figure 3).

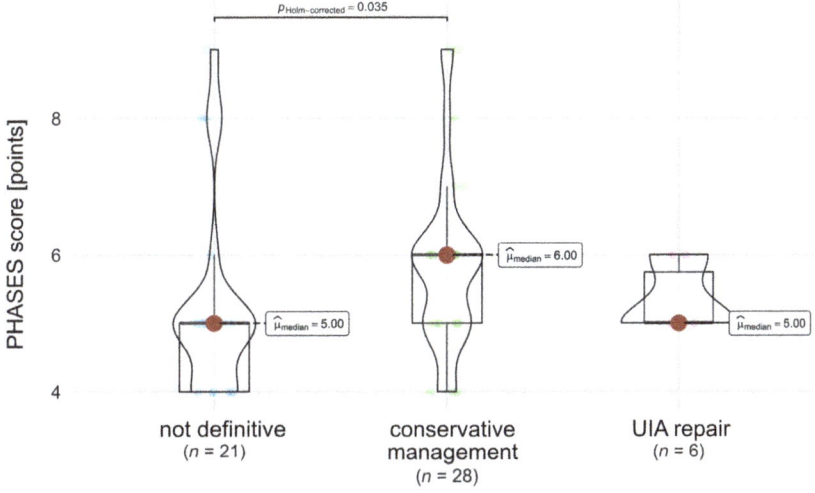

Figure 3. Comparison of PHASES scores in relation to UIATS recommendations in the observation group. A dark red dot denotes the median value, while smaller dots indicate values of individual patients.

We compared patients whom we observed following UIATS recommendations for conservative management against those whom we observed despite UIATS recommending UIA repair. Among the patients under observation in real-life management, we identified a subgroup with a UIATS UIA repair recommendation, displaying distinctive characteristics. Specifically, these patients were significantly younger [median (IQR) age of 51 (48 to 57) years old vs. median (IQR) of 72 (68 to 77) years old], had more frequent previous SAH (p = 0.025), a family history of aneurysms and/or a hemorrhage from another aneurysm in the past (p = 0.016), were more often active smokers (p = 0.016), and had multiple aneurysms significantly more often (p = 0.021, Table 4).

3.5. Treatment Group

PHASES scores in the group of patients who underwent treatment ranged from 4 to 15, with 26% (18) of them having high-risk aneurysms (PHASES score of 10 or more). According to UIATS, UIA repair was recommended for 42% (29) of patients and conservative management for 19% (13) of patients, and a recommendation was not definitive for 39% (27). The PHASES scores in these three subgroups of different UIATS recommendations among patients who underwent treatment were significantly different [Chi-squared Kruskal-Wallis = 8.12, $p = 0.017$, $\varepsilon 2 = 0.12$ (0.04; 1); Figure 4]. Notably, within the treatment group, patients with UIATS conservative management recommendations had significantly higher PHASES scores compared to other treated patients, namely those for whom UIATS recommended UIA repair or did not provide a clear recommendation ('recommendation not definitive').

Table 4. Demographic and aneurysmal information for UIATS recommending unruptured intracranial aneurysm (UIA) repair or conservative management within a group of patients with unruptured anterior communicating artery aneurysms under observation. FDR—false discovery rate, IQR—interquartile range, NA—not applicable, SAH—subarachnoid hemorrhage, UIA—unruptured intracranial aneurysm.

Parameter (Unit)	Recommendation According to UIATS		p-Value	p-Value FDR
	Conservative Management [n (%)/Median (IQR)]	UIA Repair [n (%)/Median (IQR)]		
Patients	28	6		
Age (years)	72 (68 to 77)	51 (48 to 57)	<0.001	0.008
Aneurysm size (mm)	3.94 (2.28 to 6.00)	2.10 (1.55 to 4.00)	0.094	0.12
Previous SAH for another aneurysm	1 (3.6%)	3 (50%)	0.012	0.022
Familial history	0	3 (50%)	0.003	0.014
Active smoking	5 (18%)	5 (83%)	0.005	0.014
Multiple aneurysms	6 (21%)	5 (83%)	0.008	0.019
Aspect ratio > 1.6	1.25 (0.97 to 1.75)	1.27 (0.67 to 1.60)	0.60	0.67
Size ratio > 3	1.88 (1.25 to 2.64)	0.99 (0.78 to 1.77)	0.040	0.06
Low-risk aneurysm *	28	6	NA	NA
High-risk aneurysm *	0	0		

* Evaluated with PHASES interpretation, in which a score of 10 or more assigned to the aneurysm was considered high-risk, while scores under 10 were low-risk.

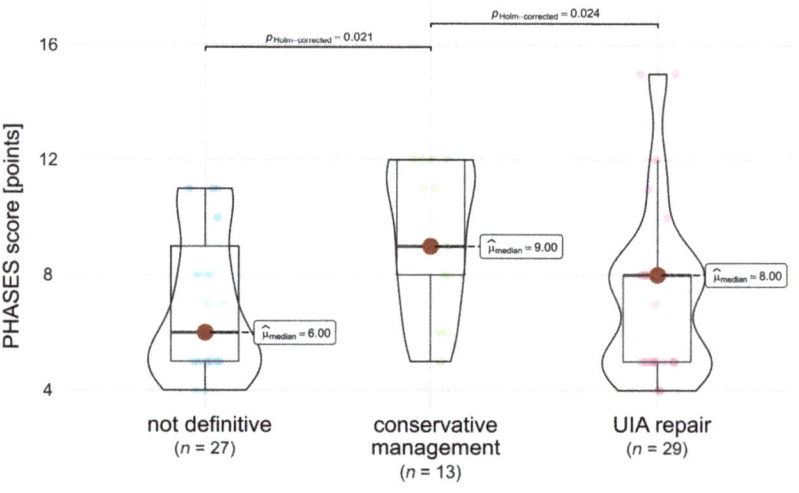

Figure 4. Comparison of PHASES scores in relation to UIATS recommendations in patients who underwent treatment. A dark red dot denotes the median value, while small dots indicate values of individual patients.

We additionally compared the aneurysms within our treatment group, distinguishing between those for which UIATS recommended UIA repair and those for which UIATS recommended conservative management. Patients with UIATS UIA repair recommendation (within the real-world treatment group) were significantly younger [median (IQR) age of 54 (48 to 58) years old vs. median (IQR) of 71 (67 to 75) years old, $p < 0.001$], were active smokers more frequently (69% vs. 0%, $p < 0.001$), but had lower PHASES scores [median (IQR) of 8 (5 to 8) vs. median (IQR) of 9 (8 to 12), $p = 0.007$], when compared against the patients within the treatment group who received UIATS observation recommendation (Table 5).

Table 5. Demographic and aneurysmal information for UIATS recommending UIA repair or conservative management within groups of patients with unruptured anterior communicating artery aneurysms who underwent treatment. FDR—false discovery rate, IQR—interquartile range, SAH—subarachnoid hemorrhage, UIA—unruptured intracranial aneurysm.

Parameter (Unit)	Recommendation According to UIATS		p-Value	p-Value FDR
	Conservative Management [n (%)/Median (IQR)]	UIA Repair [n (%)/Median (IQR)]		
Patients	13	29		
Age (years)	71 (67 to 75)	54 (48 to 58)	<0.001	<0.001
Aneurysm size (mm)	8.2 (7.5 to 10.2)	7.0 (5.5 to 9.0)	0.10	0.16
Previous SAH from another aneurysm	0	2 (6.9%)	>0.99	>0.99
Familial history	0	7 (24%)	0.079	0.16
Active smoking	0	20 (69%)	<0.001	<0.001
Multiple aneurysms	2 (15%)	13 (45%)	0.089	0.16
Multilobulated aneurysms	4 (31%)	9 (31%)	>0.99	>0.99
Aspect ratio > 1.6	1.79 (1.39 to 2.24)	1.56 (1.30 to 2.19)	0.97	>0.99
Size ratio > 3	4.32 (2.82 to 5.26)	3.12 (2.69 to 3.89)	0.059	0.16
Low-risk aneurysm *	7	23	0.16	0.22
High-risk aneurysm *	4	3		

* Evaluated with PHASES interpretation, in which a score of 10 or more assigned to the aneurysm was considered high-risk, while scores under 10 were low-risk.

3.6. Summary of the Results

As a result of our management strategy, we reserved observation only for low-risk AComA UIAs according to the PHASES score interpretation. Even so, concurrently, we treated as many as 46% (51) of low-risk aneurysms. Overall, our management was in concordance with the PHASES score interpretation in 60% of cases.

In 60% (76) of cases, UIATS recommendations were definitive, while the remaining cases were categorized as not definitive. We treated 82% (29) of cases in which UIATS recommended UIA repair and observed 68% (28) of cases for which UIATS recommended conservative management. Overall, our management was in concordance with UIATS recommendations in 46% of cases.

Surprisingly, the concordance of these two scales applied to AComA UIAs was as low as 32% (40). When comparing the UIATS and PHASES evaluations, we found that 33% (6 cases) of high-risk aneurysms (as per PHASES interpretation) received a UIATS conservative management recommendation. In as many as 39% (7) of these high-risk aneurysms, the UIATS recommendation was not definitive. On the other hand, 27% (30) of cases of low-risk aneurysms obtained a UIATS UIA repair recommendation.

In our analysis of AComA UIAs that underwent treatment, an intriguing pattern emerged when evaluating the recommendations from UIATS and PHASES. Notably, a mere 7.2% of treated AComA UIAs received a UIATS UIA repair recommendation while simultaneously being deemed high-risk according to their PHASES interpretation. The majority of treated aneurysms (61%) fell into either the high-risk category based on their PHASES interpretation, or received a UIA repair recommendation from UIATS.

4. Discussion

The AComA complex is a prevalent site for UIAs, constituting up to 33% of cases. A number of studies underscore its elevated risk of rupture, as indicated by a meta-analysis reporting a 2.51 times higher risk for AComA aneurysms compared to those in other anterior circulation sites [15,16]. Moreover, small AComA UIAs have been reported to bear a similar risk of rupture to posterior circulation aneurysms [17]. The conjunction and synergy of these two features established the foundation for distinguishing AComA aneurysms from other locations within the anterior circulation in our studies.

The PHASES score emerged from a collaborative effort among researchers from diverse institutions, originating in a large international study that synthesized data from individual patient records and aneurysm databases [9]. Developed by analyzing various risk factors and their associations with aneurysm rupture, the PHASES score serves as a tool for clinicians to estimate rupture risk in UIAs based on individual patient characteristics [18].

The UIATS recommendations, representing a consensus effort among researchers, were developed through a comprehensive analysis of data from various sources, including individual patient records and aneurysm databases [10]. These guidelines provide clinicians with evidence-based insights for managing UIAs [19].

4.1. UIATS Recommendations

In our investigation, we identified instances where the recommendations provided by UIATS were not clearly delineated. This raises concerns about the suitability of using UIATS in isolation. Notably, patients who were observed in real-life settings more frequently received a UIATS recommendation for conservative management than a recommendation for UIA repair. Nevertheless, 11% of these patients (6) were recommended to undergo UIA repair. This subset of patients, receiving a UIATS UIA repair recommendation and who remained under observation in real life, exhibited distinct characteristics—they were notably younger, had a higher incidence of familial history related to aneurysms or prior hemorrhages from another aneurysm, were more likely to smoke, and presented with multiple aneurysms. Interestingly, the aneurysms in the observation group with a UIATS UIA repair recommendation were very small (median size 2.1 mm), even when compared to those in the subgroup receiving a UIATS conservative management recommendation, although this difference was not statistically significant. This persistent UIA repair recommendation was noteworthy, particularly in light of three points favoring conservative management, which were justified by the aneurysm's complexity arising from a very small diameter (<3 mm).

It is worth noting that, within the treatment group, significantly older patients consistently received UIATS conservative management recommendations. This feature of UIATS, evident in patients who underwent treatment in our real-life scenario, harmonizes with the study by Rutledge et al. [20]. The researchers reported that UIATS tends to underestimate the risk of hemorrhage in older patients. Moreover, older patients are more severely affected by aneurysmal hemorrhage [21,22]. This emphasizes the need for a critical evaluation of UIATS recommendations in older populations, recognizing the potential underestimation of hemorrhage risk and the heightened severity of aneurysmal hemorrhage in this demographic.

4.2. PHASES Scores

Although patients who underwent preventive aneurysm repair had significantly higher PHASES scores, we treated almost half (46%, 51) of patients with low–risk aneurysms (according to PHASES interpretation). An additional analysis of these cases unveiled that the vast majority (96%, 49) harbored at least one type A risk factor, and two-thirds (66.7%, 34) had two type A risk factors, according to Chalouhi et al. [23]. The remaining 4% of patients had one type A risk factor and one type B factor, which advocates for treatment, according to the researcher's algorithm. In our management approach, we did not observe any high-risk aneurysms (as per PHASES interpretation).

4.3. UIATS and PHASES Comparison

As presented in the summary of the results, a notable discordance between PHASES and UIATS persists in AComA UIAs: every third high-risk aneurysm, as per PHASES interpretation, received a UIA repair recommendation according to UIATS. Overall, the concordance of these scales was 32%. It would be reasonable to assume that using more tools should help with daily clinical practice, but our results show that the use of these scales did not make decision-making simpler, instead adding to the confusion on what to do. In certain scenarios, it appears likely that UIATS recommends conservative management for high-risk aneurysms (as per PHASES) due to the consideration of treatment-related risks. Unfortunately, an analogous explanation for why UIATS recommends UIA repair for low-risk aneurysms in certain cases remains elusive.

What is more, we observed two unusual findings - one within the observation group, and another within the treatment group. Firstly, among patients under observation, the subgroup with a UIATS conservative management recommendation had significantly higher PHASES scores compared to patients with a "not definitive" recommendation. The apparent contradiction in this finding may be attributed to the objective of UIATS construction, which considers not only aneurysm characteristics but also the inherent risks of treatment. Such a comprehensive approach may lead to a final recommendation favoring conservative management, despite apparent higher aneurysm risks depicted by relatively higher PHASES scores.

Secondly, within the treatment group, patients with UIATS conservative management recommendations had significantly higher PHASES scores compared to other treated patients, specifically those for whom UIATS recommended UIA repair or did not provide a clear recommendation. This apparent paradox may be simply explained by our management approach, wherein patients with high-risk aneurysms (as per PHASES interpretation) were qualified for treatment, regardless of other associated risks indicated in the UIATS recommendations. In essence, our decision to opt for patient treatment was influenced by the recommendation of only one of the scales.

4.4. Limitations of Aneurysm Scale Use

Scales intended to forecast the risk of aneurysm hemorrhage or offer clinical guidance are not commonly integrated into clinical practice [24]. Additionally, these scales suffer from a notable deficit of prospective evaluation, a crucial element requisite for establishing a robust scientific basis to support their widespread implementation [19]. On the contrary, there are a number of studies that have been critical of using these scales. Ravindra et al. concluded that UIATS recommended the overtreatment of unruptured aneurysms [19]. When analyzing ruptured aneurysms, Rutledge et al. found that applying UIATS to elderly patients would have led to their undertreatment, a problem not observed in younger populations [20]. Furthermore, Hernandez-Duran et al. found that the sensitivity of UIATS in detecting high-risk aneurysms in ruptured aneurysm cases was low [25]. On the contrary, Feghali et al. showed that UIATS demonstrated good concordance with real-world practice [26].

A major shortcoming of UIATS was recently reported by Stumpo et al. [5]. The researchers claimed that UIATS would have failed to recommend UIA repair in 72.6% of patients whose aneurysms eventually ruptured. Additionally, Molenberg et al. reported poor performance of UIATS in predicting aneurysm growth or rupture [27].

4.5. Study Limitations

This study possesses inherent limitations attributed to its retrospective design, a relatively modest sample size, and single-center focus. While the latter introduces a degree of subjectivity to the patient group, management processes, and results evaluation, we contend that this limitation offers unique strengths within the specific context of our investigation.

The homogeneity observed in the evaluated AComA UIAs, coupled with the consistent approach to management decisions (albeit with some adjustments over time) resulting from our single-center methodology, provides a distinctive advantage. This homogeneity facilitates direct comparisons, enabling the derivation of meaningful conclusions—a feat that might prove challenging in a multicenter, retrospective study design with potentially increased variability in patient populations and management practices. The inclusion of numerous centers may introduce additional confounding factors, complicating the interpretation of results.

Furthermore, as previously noted in our earlier publication, a subset of patients from external medical facilities qualified for observation. However, their data are not incorporated into our databases [8]. Consequently, the reported number of patients under observation in this study represents only a fraction of the total AComA UIAs under observation, excluding those managed at external hospitals and outpatient clinics. This omission emphasizes the necessity for cautious generalization of our findings to broader patient populations.

Finally, an important limitation of our study lies in the use of the PHASES score interpretation. Following the approach outlined by Stumpo et al., we categorized aneurysms into high- and low-risk groups, subsequently assigning them to treatment and observation, respectively [11]. It is crucial to acknowledge this methodology when interpreting the results of our investigation. However, the necessity for some degree of generalization, including the use of, at times, arbitrary cutoffs, is recognized to facilitate evaluation in a broader context.

4.6. Final Remarks and Future Directions

Assessing the concordance of aneurysm management with PHASES scores proves challenging, as PHASES scoring primarily estimates the risk of hemorrhage rather than guiding aneurysm management. As per the European Stroke Organisation guidelines, preventive aneurysm repair is recommended for individuals with a 5-year risk of aneurysm rupture, as this surpasses the risks associated with preventive treatment [28]. The impact of implementation of the PHASES score in aneurysm management was evaluated by Hollands et al. [29]. The researchers found that out of two examined centers, one did not change its previous practice, while the other began to qualify less aneurysms for treatment.

In our management, we disqualified high-risk aneurysms from observation, and a substantial number of low-risk aneurysms were treated (as assessed with PHASES interpretation). This finding aligns with the observations of Longnon et al., who reported that PHASES did not identify the majority of patients as being at a high or intermediate risk of rupture [6]. Hilditch et al. reported comparable results [30].

The second noteworthy finding is the divergence in suggestions between PHASES and UIATS in numerous cases. While this initial discrepancy may complicate decision-making, a potential strategy could involve using the PHASES scale to estimate the risk of hemorrhage. Subsequently, if an aneurysm is identified as high risk, the UIATS scale could serve as a more refined tool to strike a balance between the risk of rupture and the risk of treatment. Such a scheme necessitates future prospective evaluation.

Furthermore, prospective multicenter studies, utilizing established frameworks like UIATS and PHASES, are crucial and much needed for advancing our understanding of AComA UIAs. A collaborative, prospective approach in properly designed multicenter studies would enhance the generalizability of findings, capturing diverse patient demographics and management practices. These studies should focus on elucidating natural history and risk factors of UIAs, as well as establishing a consensus on optimal management and the usefulness of clinical scales. Moreover, crucial additional outcomes to consider encompass the real-world morbidity associated with interventions for UIAs and their consequential impact on patients' quality of life. The use of standardized assessment tools ensures a consistent framework, contributing to evidence-based guidelines for improved clinical decision-making.

5. Conclusions

Over two thirds of the evaluations in the AComA UIA group yielded discordant suggestions between PHASES and UIATS assessments. This underscores that therapeutic decisions continue to be primarily influenced by the center's experience, individual assessments, and patient preferences. Recognizing the shortcomings of currently used scales, future prospective studies are needed to refine and validate decision-making strategies for managing UIAs. This may involve exploring alternative applications of current scales and developing new ones tailored to specific patients and aneurysms.

Supplementary Materials: The following supporting information can be downloaded at: https://www.mdpi.com/article/10.3390/jcm13030789/s1, Supplementary Table S1. Distribution of the PHASES scores across UIATS recommendations in patients with unruptured anterior communicating artery aneurysms. UIA—unruptured intracranial aneurysm.

Author Contributions: Conceptualization, K.W., L.P. and P.K.; methodology, K.W., L.P., P.K. and S.K.; software, S.K.; validation, P.K., L.P., E.M. and K.W.; formal analysis, P.K., L.P., K.W., E.M. and S.K.; investigation, K.W., S.K. and A.M.; resources, K.W., L.P., E.M. and A.M.; data curation, K.W. and L.P.; writing—original draft preparation, K.W. and L.P.; writing—review and editing, L.P. and P.K.; visualization, K.W.; supervision, P.K. and A.M.; project administration, L.P. All authors have read and agreed to the published version of the manuscript.

Funding: This research received no external funding.

Institutional Review Board Statement: This study was conducted in accordance with the Declaration of Helsinki and approved by the Bioethics Committee of the Medical University of Warsaw (Approval code AKBE/121/2023 Approved date 3 April 2023).

Informed Consent Statement: Patient consent was waived by the Bioethics Committee of the Medical University of Warsaw due to the retrospective character of the study and participants' anonymity.

Data Availability Statement: The data presented in this study are available on request from the corresponding author after acceptance of all the co-authors.

Acknowledgments: The authors would like to thank Andrew Tuson for his language editing help in preparing the manuscript.

Conflicts of Interest: The authors declare no conflict of interest.

References

1. Laukka, D.; Kivelev, J.; Rahi, M.; Vahlberg, T.; Paturi, J.; Rinne, J.; Hirvonen, J. Detection Rates and Trends of Asymptomatic Unruptured Intracranial Aneurysms From 2005 to 2019. *Neurosurgery* **2023**, *94*, 297–306. [CrossRef] [PubMed]
2. Khorasanizadeh, M.; Pettersson, S.D.; Maglinger, B.; Garcia, A.; Wang, S.J.; Ogilvy, C.S. Trends in the Size of Treated Unruptured Intracranial Aneurysms over 35 Years. *J. Neurosurg.* **2023**, *139*, 1328–1338. [CrossRef] [PubMed]
3. Pettersson, S.D.; Khorasanizadeh, M.; Maglinger, B.; Garcia, A.; Wang, S.J.; Taussky, P.; Ogilvy, C.S. Trends in the Age of Patients Treated for Unruptured Intracranial Aneurysms from 1990 to 2020. *World Neurosurg.* **2023**, *178*, 233–240.e13. [CrossRef] [PubMed]
4. Sturiale, C.L.; Stumpo, V.; Ricciardi, L.; Trevisi, G.; Valente, I.; D'Arrigo, S.; Latour, K.; Barbone, P.; Albanese, A. Retrospective Application of Risk Scores to Ruptured Intracranial Aneurysms: Would They Have Predicted the Risk of Bleeding? *Neurosurg. Rev.* **2021**, *44*, 1655–1663. [CrossRef] [PubMed]
5. Stumpo, V.; Latour, K.; Trevisi, G.; Valente, I.; D'Arrigo, S.; Mangiola, A.; Olivi, A.; Sturiale, C.L. Retrospective Application of UIATS Recommendations to a Multicenter Cohort of Ruptured Intracranial Aneurysms: How It Would Have Oriented the Treatment Choices? *World Neurosurg.* **2021**, *147*, e262–e271. [CrossRef]
6. Lognon, P.; Gariel, F.; Marnat, G.; Darcourt, J.; Constant Dit Beaufils, P.; Burel, J.; Shotar, E.; Hak, J.F.; Fauché, C.; Kerleroux, B.; et al. Prospective Assessment of Aneurysmal Rupture Risk Scores in Patients with Subarachnoid Hemorrhage: A Multicentric Cohort. *Neuroradiology* **2022**, *64*, 2363–2371. [CrossRef]
7. Pagiola, I.; Mihalea, C.; Caroff, J.; Ikka, L.; Chalumeau, V.; Iacobucci, M.; Ozanne, A.; Gallas, S.; Marques, M.; Nalli, D.; et al. The PHASES Score: To Treat or Not to Treat? Retrospective Evaluation of the Risk of Rupture of Intracranial Aneurysms in Patients with Aneurysmal Subarachnoid Hemorrhage. *J. Neuroradiol.* **2020**, *47*, 349–352. [CrossRef]
8. Wójtowicz, K.; Przepiorka, L.; Kujawski, S.; Marchel, A.; Kunert, P. Unruptured Anterior Communicating Artery Aneurysms: Management Strategy and Results of a Single-Center Experience. *J. Clin. Med.* **2023**, *12*, 4619. [CrossRef]

9. Greving, J.P.; Wermer, M.J.H.; Brown, R.D.; Morita, A.; Juvela, S.; Yonekura, M.; Ishibashi, T.; Torner, J.C.; Nakayama, T.; Rinkel, G.J.E.; et al. Development of the PHASES Score for Prediction of Risk of Rupture of Intracranial Aneurysms: A Pooled Analysis of Six Prospective Cohort Studies. *Lancet Neurol.* **2014**, *13*, 59–66. [CrossRef] [PubMed]
10. Etminan, N.; Brown, R.D.; Beseoglu, K.; Juvela, S.; Raymond, J.; Morita, A.; Torner, J.C.; Derdeyn, C.P.; Raabe, A.; Mocco, J.; et al. The Unruptured Intracranial Aneurysm Treatment Score: A Multidisciplinary Consensus. *Neurology* **2015**, *85*, 881–889. [CrossRef] [PubMed]
11. Stumpo, V.; Latour, K.; Trevisi, G.; Valente, I.; D'Arrigo, S.; Olivi, A.; Sturiale, C.L. Comparison between Rupture/Growth Risk Scores and Treatment Recommendation Scores Application to Aneurysmal Subarachnoid Hemorrhage Patients: A Multicenter Cross-Reliability Assessment Study. *J. Clin. Neurosci.* **2022**, *99*, 359–366. [CrossRef]
12. *The Jamovi Project*, Version 2.3; Jamovi: Sydney, Australia, 2023.
13. R Core Team. *R: A Language and Environment for Statistical Computing*; R Foundation for Statistical Computing: Vienna, Austria, 2021.
14. Patil, I. Ggstatsplot: Ggplot2 Based Plots with Statistical Details. 2021. Available online: https://indrajeetpatil.github.io/ggstatsplot/ (accessed on 24 January 2024).
15. Mira, J.M.S.; Costa, F.A.D.O.; Horta, B.L.; Fabião, O.M. Risk of Rupture in Unruptured Anterior Communicating Artery Aneurysms: Meta-Analysis of Natural History Studies. *Surg. Neurol.* **2006**, *66* (Suppl. S3), S12–S19; discussion S19. [CrossRef] [PubMed]
16. Juvela, S. Outcome of Patients with Multiple Intracranial Aneurysms after Subarachnoid Hemorrhage and Future Risk of Rupture of Unruptured Aneurysm. *J. Clin. Med.* **2021**, *10*, 1712. [CrossRef] [PubMed]
17. Bijlenga, P.; Ebeling, C.; Jaegersberg, M.; Summers, P.; Rogers, A.; Waterworth, A.; Iavindrasana, J.; Macho, J.; Pereira, V.M.; Bukovics, P.; et al. Risk of Rupture of Small Anterior Communicating Artery Aneurysms Is Similar to Posterior Circulation Aneurysms. *Stroke* **2013**, *44*, 3018–3026. [CrossRef] [PubMed]
18. Bijlenga, P.; Gondar, R.; Schilling, S.; Morel, S.; Hirsch, S.; Cuony, J.; Corniola, M.-V.; Perren, F.; Rüfenacht, D.; Schaller, K. PHASES Score for the Management of Intracranial Aneurysm: A Cross-Sectional Population-Based Retrospective Study. *Stroke* **2017**, *48*, 2105–2112. [CrossRef]
19. Ravindra, V.M.; de Havenon, A.; Gooldy, T.C.; Scoville, J.; Guan, J.; Couldwell, W.T.; Taussky, P.; MacDonald, J.D.; Schmidt, R.H.; Park, M.S. Validation of the Unruptured Intracranial Aneurysm Treatment Score: Comparison with Real-World Cerebrovascular Practice. *J. Neurosurg.* **2018**, *129*, 100–106. [CrossRef] [PubMed]
20. Rutledge, C.; Raper, D.M.S.; Jonzzon, S.; Raygor, K.P.; Pereira, M.P.; Winkler, E.A.; Zhang, L.; Lawton, M.T.; Abla, A.A. Sensitivity of the Unruptured Intracranial Aneurysm Treatment Score (UIATS) in the Elderly: Retrospective Analysis of Ruptured Aneurysms. *World Neurosurg.* **2021**, *152*, e673–e677. [CrossRef] [PubMed]
21. Goldberg, J.; Schoeni, D.; Mordasini, P.; Z'Graggen, W.; Gralla, J.; Raabe, A.; Beck, J.; Fung, C. Survival and Outcome after Poor-Grade Aneurysmal Subarachnoid Hemorrhage in Elderly Patients. *Stroke* **2018**, *49*, 2883–2889. [CrossRef]
22. Lanzino, G.; Kassell, N.F.; Germanson, T.P.; Kongable, G.L.; Truskowski, L.L.; Torner, J.C.; Jane, J.A. Age and Outcome after Aneurysmal Subarachnoid Hemorrhage: Why Do Older Patients Fare Worse? *J. Neurosurg.* **1996**, *85*, 410–418. [CrossRef]
23. Chalouhi, N.; Dumont, A.S.; Randazzo, C.; Tjoumakaris, S.; Gonzalez, L.F.; Rosenwasser, R.; Jabbour, P. Management of Incidentally Discovered Intracranial Vascular Abnormalities. *Neurosurg. Focus* **2011**, *31*, E1. [CrossRef]
24. Sanchez, S.; Miller, J.M.; Samaniego, E.A. Clinical Scales in Aneurysm Rupture Prediction. *Stroke Vasc. Interv. Neurol.* **2023**, *4*, e000625. [CrossRef]
25. Hernández-Durán, S.; Mielke, D.; Rohde, V.; Malinova, V. Is the Unruptured Intracranial Aneurysm Treatment Score (UIATS) Sensitive Enough to Detect Aneurysms at Risk of Rupture? *Neurosurg. Rev.* **2021**, *44*, 987–993. [CrossRef]
26. Feghali, J.; Gami, A.; Caplan, J.M.; Tamargo, R.J.; McDougall, C.G.; Huang, J. Management of Unruptured Intracranial Aneurysms: Correlation of UIATS, ELAPSS, and PHASES with Referral Center Practice. *Neurosurg. Rev.* **2021**, *44*, 1625–1633. [CrossRef]
27. Molenberg, R.; Aalbers, M.W.; Mazuri, A.; Luijckx, G.J.; Metzemaekers, J.D.M.; Groen, R.J.M.; Uyttenboogaart, M.; van Dijk, J.M.C. The Unruptured Intracranial Aneurysm Treatment Score as a Predictor of Aneurysm Growth or Rupture. *Eur. J. Neurol.* **2021**, *28*, 837–843. [CrossRef]
28. Etminan, N.; de Sousa, D.A.; Tiseo, C.; Bourcier, R.; Desal, H.; Lindgren, A.; Koivisto, T.; Netuka, D.; Peschillo, S.; Lémeret, S.; et al. European Stroke Organisation (ESO) Guidelines on Management of Unruptured Intracranial Aneurysms. *Eur. Stroke J.* **2022**, *7*, LXXXI-CVI. [CrossRef] [PubMed]
29. Hollands, L.J.; Vergouwen, M.D.I.; Greving, J.P.; Wermer, M.J.H.; Rinkel, G.J.E.; Algra, A.M. Management Decisions on Unruptured Intracranial Aneurysms before and after Implementation of the PHASES Score. *J. Neurol. Sci.* **2021**, *422*, 117319. [CrossRef] [PubMed]
30. Hilditch, C.A.; Brinjikji, W.; Tsang, A.; Nicholson, P.; Kostynskyy, A.; Tymianski, M.; Krings, T.; Radovanovic, I.; Pereira, V. Application of PHASES and ELAPSS Scores to Ruptured Cerebral Aneurysms: How Many Would Have Been Conservatively Managed? *J. Neurosurg. Sci.* **2021**, *65*, 33–37. [CrossRef] [PubMed]

Disclaimer/Publisher's Note: The statements, opinions and data contained in all publications are solely those of the individual author(s) and contributor(s) and not of MDPI and/or the editor(s). MDPI and/or the editor(s) disclaim responsibility for any injury to people or property resulting from any ideas, methods, instructions or products referred to in the content.

MDPI
St. Alban-Anlage 66
4052 Basel
Switzerland
www.mdpi.com

Journal of Clinical Medicine Editorial Office
E-mail: jcm@mdpi.com
www.mdpi.com/journal/jcm

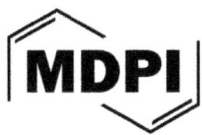

Disclaimer/Publisher's Note: The statements, opinions and data contained in all publications are solely those of the individual author(s) and contributor(s) and not of MDPI and/or the editor(s). MDPI and/or the editor(s) disclaim responsibility for any injury to people or property resulting from any ideas, methods, instructions or products referred to in the content.

www.ingramcontent.com/pod-product-compliance
Lightning Source LLC
LaVergne TN
LVHW070558100526
838202LV00012B/500